I
Always
Wanted To
Be A Dad:
Men
Without
Children

Robert Nurden

First published in the UK in August 2023

Text copyright © 2023 Robert Nurden

Edited by Rosalyn Scott

Proofreading by Annie Deakins, Proofnow

Cover and book design by Berenice Howard-Smith, Hello Lovely and The Full Stop

ISBN: 978-1-8384477-3-1

Printed in the UK

Image credits: with thanks to the contributors for their images, page 54 Alexey Fedorenko, *Shutterstock*. Other images author's own.

robertnurden.com

Acknowledgements

My thanks to Sue Rowlands, Berenice Howard-Smith,
Rosalyn Scott, Dr Robin A Hadley, Jody Day, Jessica Hepburn,
Stephanie Joy Phillips, Andy Harrod, Michael Hughes, Annie
Kirby, Rob Hutchings, Guy Shennan, Mike Carter, Mark
H. Mark Massé, John Lent, Kevin Scanlan, Denise Felkin
and the many other people who contributed to this book.

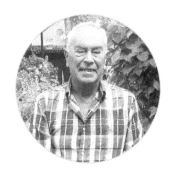

About the Author

ROBERT NURDEN WAS a feature writer and sub-editor for the *Guardian*, *Independent* and *Daily Telegraph*, as well as many other national newspapers and magazines. He published his first book, *Between Heaven and Earth: A Journey with My Grandfather*, in 2021. He teaches English and Journalism and lives in east London.

To My Unborn Child

Foreword

IT IS AN honour to write a foreword to Robert's book, *I Always Wanted To Be A Dad: Men Without Children*. We first met Robert online a couple of years ago, when he discussed capturing childless men's experiences for a book. Robert's original idea has flourished into this brave book you now hold, which highlights not only his own voice, but also the voices of other men who wanted to be a dad.

Childless grief is full of intangible losses and moments, which are intensely personal and very often invisible to those around us. And at times to ourselves. Robert courageously untangles some of the messiness and complexity of the reality of not being a dad and living without children. His experiences are offered clipped, disjointed – this staccato style reflects the reality. It hits you. Again. And again. For coming to terms with not being a dad is not a tidy or linear process. It is messy, painful and complex.

Robert gives substance to our invisible losses through openly sharing his feelings and thoughts and aligning his experiences with those of other childless men. Through his snapshots, he creates space for engagement; providing room for the experiences to breathe and leave the page. For the reader to connect through their own experiences, combatting feelings of 'it's just me', in the creation of new narratives on this journey together.

The experiences Robert shares are particularly powerful as they reflect how everyday situations become deeply unsettling for men without children, as well as revealing the depths of a man's desire to be a dad and the paths considered. While he opens himself up to judgement and comment through not shying away from any aspect of his journey, for us childless men, he has become a trailblazer.

Ultimately, this is a tremendously brave book as Robert has shaken off societal norms through his honest, emotive and generous writing. His writing reflects a path that moves towards acceptance of a situation he never expected. An acceptance that is uneasy, but also suggests to us men who wanted to be a dad, that a meaningful, purposeful and joyful life is possible.

Andy Harrod & Michael Hughes

Founders of The Childless Men's Community

Praise for *I Always Wanted To Be A Dad: Men Without Children*

I love this book. With breath-taking honesty and eloquence, Robert Nurden has articulated the life and times of a man who is childless not by choice. It is a powerful reminder that, in terms of fertility and parenthood, women have dominated the discourse. It's time for men to be heard. The highest praise I can give this brave and brilliant book is that Robert made me want to lean forward and listen.
Jessica Hepburn, author of 21 Miles and The Pursuit of Motherhood

Robert Nurden's book is an extremely moving account of his experience of unwanted childlessness. He guides us through the deeply personal thoughts and feelings about fatherhood and the intricacies of his relationships. He deepens his multi-layered emotional journey by including the voices of other circumstantial childless men.
Dr Robin A. Hadley, author of How Is a Man Supposed to Be a Man?

A much-needed autobiographical exploration from a childless-by-circumstance man as he unravels how and why his desire for fatherhood was thwarted. Tender, illuminating, angry, surprising and deeply vulnerable, it shows that behind every man without children is a complex, and until now, untold story, and as deserving of empathy and respect as those of childless women.
Jody Day, founder of Gateway Women and author of Living the Life Unexpected

I loved this book. It is filled with humour, heartache, and the hard-won battle of accepting painful circumstances. I felt like Robert and I were talking face-to-face. A must-read.
Rob Hutchings, author of Downriver Nomad

This is an important and timely exploration of the neglected topic of male childlessness. Both moving and brutally honest, Robert Nurden's book – which combines his own memoir of childlessness with testimony from other childless men – shines a light on the loneliness, grief and exclusion experienced by men who dreamt of fatherhood but never had children. An essential addition to the literature dealing with childlessness.

Annie Kirby, author of The Hollow Sea

Taking on the raw and undiscussed topic of involuntary male childlessness, this ground-breaking and necessary book is full of grief, regret and despair. And then the upward trajectory of its ending is all the more powerful, as we are left with a sense of possibility, hope and life. A wonderful book.

Guy Shennan, therapist and author of Solution-Focused Practice

Warmth and humour mixed with grief, regret and hard-hitting reality combine to create a compelling read, as Robert shares his thoughts on arriving at a destination he never expected or wanted.

Stephanie Joy Phillips, founder of World Childless Week

A timely and valuable contribution to a subject little talked about, let alone written about. Let's hope it helps to get childless men talking more openly about what can be a devastating hole in their lives.

Mike Carter, author of One Man and His Bike

Robert Nurden has written a heartfelt book about being a childless man, reflecting on the pain, regret and questions facing someone in his twilight years. What's most important is, as Nurden shows, to make peace with life and its mysteries.

Mark H. Massé, author of Nobody's Father

A grounded, human look at an issue that is ignored in our culture. This is a compelling, at times brutal, but moving and triumphant examination of a complex human puzzle.

John Lent, poet and author of Navigating the River of No Return

Contents

Introduction

IT IS NO surprise that the issue of unwanted childlessness is almost always seen through the eyes of women. After all, they are exclusively responsible for childbirth and the greater part of early years' care. But men often long to have children of their own too and the resulting hurt when life doesn't bring them the family they craved can hit just as hard.

I am one of those men and this book is a collection of my thoughts and feelings as I confront my childless reality. Other men in the same situation add their voices to show it's time for this neglected problem to be recognised.

A warning: this is no easy read. You will encounter anger, pain and despair. The despair of the man who has remained childless despite a burning desire to be otherwise. You will come across mistakes and life courses not going to plan. Sometimes the fault will lie with the individual and the choices he has made; sometimes the cause is just bad luck, poor timing or ill judgement; sometimes it is for medical reasons such as infertility or for a complex combination of factors beyond the man's control. This is a stark record of men's lives going wrong.

The content reflects my own position, which is that of being childless by circumstance, rather than being childless due to infertility. I have focused on those who are childless not by choice, rather than those who have taken a positive decision to remain that way. Alongside the pieces authored by me here lie the testimonies of other men and their countless reasons for being childless. Many of them belong to the Facebook group The Childless Men's Community, which offers support to men around the world. Others are friends of mine. I hope that this largely unacknowledged state, in which 25 per cent of men over 42 find themselves childless, may finally be understood.

The main part of this book is composed of short, unstructured chapters about my own life that are deliberately rough, edgy and raw. The stories have no tidy endings. Characters are left behind, never to be seen or heard of again. In many ways this is an uncontrolled scream, with me and others shouting loudly in an empty room. This is the only way I could write it and I needed to share it. Nor is there any neat, therapeutic conclusion: I distrust those. I am no moral crusader. It would simply be dishonest to fashion a shaky panacea from this wreckage of damaged hopes and dreams.

But − and it's a big but − the narrative does slowly move in a positive direction, with its arc curving away from hopelessness. It follows the commonly accepted trajectory of grief from anger to acceptance. So, as the going gets rough, I implore you to hold on: the gloom lifts and a brighter horizon beckons. There is even some solace. It's a bit of a mystery where exactly that lifting of despair comes from. I didn't plan it and this book grew organically. And I really wanted to share that with you, as such change can be wonderful and profound precisely because it is so unexpected.

Perhaps I spoke too emphatically of pain and I may have misled you. I do, in fact, manage to calmly reflect on the issue of childlessness and so do the other men. There is some analysis and wistful, nostalgic regret, along with returns to a past that helped shape the present along lines we never wanted. There are even wisps of contentment. And, at the end, there is an awkward acceptance, a faltering resolution. Which itself may be the start of another, very different journey.

All names appearing in the chapters have been changed to protect people's privacy.

All Aboard the Pronatalism Express

The Train

THEY GOT ON at West Ham station and sat opposite me. I'd started my journey on the Jubilee Line at Stratford and was going into central London to see some exhibition; I forget what it was.

They were a happy Saturday morning family: Mum, Dad, two kids, about 10 and eight. Where were they going? The Science Museum? Madame Tussauds? The Changing of the Guard? McDonald's?

It was a weekend scene: a flurry of activity, the snatching back of mobile phones, the pulling of faces, the admonitory glances from a parent when they thought one of the kids had transgressed Tube train etiquette.

It was a display of anarchic freedom acted out in the calm waters of confident parental love. It was playing up, but within boundaries. Boundaries which everyone was familiar with. My partner and I were drawn into this exhibition of generational jousting. We glanced at each other and smiled. The smile stayed on our lips as we looked across the gangway at the mother. She acknowledged us and produced a faint, watery grin.

The train entered the tunnel just after Canning Town and then the magic broke. Something in me snapped. What I had been watching was no longer an enchanting performance. Now all I could see was a family of four. And all I could feel was a knife plunged into my ribs. I felt sick, leaned forward and clenched my teeth. One arm lifted without purpose and fell again into my lap. I stared at the advertisements. One was for online dating. Another for hair gel. A third asked customers to continue to wear a face mask.

'Are you OK?' my partner asked.

'Sorry, I can't take this anymore. I've got to move.'

She sighed. 'Not again? You did this last week.'

'I know. I can't help it.'

'Don't you think it's time you accepted the fact that every time you travel on the Tube you're going to see families?'

'Yes, of course it's *time*.' I sarcastically echoed her choice of words. I got up and walked down the carriage, leaving it up to her whether she followed or stayed put. Luckily, she followed me. And I never saw that family again.

I was breathing heavily. My heart was beating hard. Beads of sweat had broken out on my brow. I sat down in an empty seat and she joined me, taking my hand and squeezing it. She leaned across and kissed me on the lips. God, I was lucky to have her.

'Sorry, but I just can't stand it. Staring me in the face like that, mocking me for all that I haven't achieved.'

The Dinner Party

AS USUAL, ANNE, when she and her husband came to dinner, told us about the family, more specifically her three children. They were, of course, all perfect – 'blooming' and doing terribly well. One was a dentist, another training to be a chartered surveyor and the third – I forget: my brain had atrophied by that point. The speech was delivered from deep inside the cocoon of a mother's certainty, from on high, from a pedestal that dominated the landscape around it, acres of unchallenged emotional territory as far as the eye could see.

She was standing at the mouth of her lair, protecting her young ones (no longer young, if truth be told) from any scavenging enemies, or from anyone who questioned one iota of worth or value they may possess. Nor was there any realisation of the impact that her presentation may have had on the childless adults present.

Here, then, is unchallenged, domestic pronatalism. The absolute inability to acknowledge any other way, let alone to listen to what it might have to say. To such people, and that is most parents, adults without children are merely experiencing a painless absence. It's unfortunate, but there's no need to dwell on it.

After she left, as soon as the door closed, I choked and gasped. The utter helplessness and impotence of it all. Wracked by the thought that it needn't have been like this. The tearing thought that I could have been – should have been – a father. I crumpled into a sobbing, heaving heap on the kitchen floor where I had ended up, instead of washing up the dishes. My grief was huge and wide. And it was stoked by the fact that no one at the dinner party had asked me about my life. Having no children is equal to having no life worth talking about.

Family Values

THE NUCLEAR FAMILY is a pillar of society that is seen as being beyond criticism. It's an established structure in which its paid-up members feel safe being part of. They belong. 'Family values' and 'hard-working families' are the mantras that ring from 21st century Mammon's steeples and turrets, summoning the great and good to ceremonies of societal rectitude.

The family is the staple of safe conversation. Men and women can talk about their children in the knowledge that they will not be seriously challenged. Having a family ticks the required boxes. In a world of shifting allegiances, lies and echo chambers, it provides a sense of belonging.

I need hardly say that I'm talking about the heteronormative family here – not solo mums, gay couples or even unhappy families in which children may be taken into care. They, too, can all feel 'apart'.

So, by inventing the collocation 'Family Totalitarianism', I am venturing into dangerous territory. I am very much the David to the powerful Goliath collective of fathers, mothers and kids. Oh yes, and cousins, uncles, aunts, grandfathers and grandmothers. My position is pretty untenable. But there's nothing I can do about that.

Jan

EVERY DAY I grieve for not being a father. It's the biggest loss of my life and it makes me feel so sad. The grief is mixed with anger, frustration, unfairness, hopelessness and envy. I talk to very few people about it, not even my closest family. I find people would have more understanding if you had cancer.

Jason

I AM STILL coming to terms with never having children from my sperm and what that means to me, but that pales when comparing to not having children at all. I think it's something that I will be dealing with for the rest of my life. Grieving for a life that hasn't been born is how I would describe not being a father. Instead of grieving for a life lost – thinking about the moments enjoyed together – it's [about] grieving for moments that could have been.

Sheffield Blues

I HAD KNOWN for a long time that a good friend of mine had gone out with my ex-girlfriend in 1974 and that he'd ended up marrying her. There were no complaints. After all, it was me who finished with her, not the other way round. I left Herefordshire after my teacher training course was over and went to work as a journalist in Sussex.

I remember we said goodbye on the bridge over the River Wye in Hereford. It was sad, undoubtedly. I was hitching to London and needed to get on the road. I turned away but Julia ran after me and held me once more. We did see each other again. Once or twice, she travelled down to Sussex and stayed the weekend.

I sometimes wondered whether I had made the right decision; I even had some regrets. I won't say there weren't moments of reflection.

But Julia and I wouldn't really have been suited for the long haul. I had so much I still wanted to do as an independent man. Our aims and ambitions would have clashed.

Later, soon after Martin and Julia started going out, I was driving up Charing Cross Road in London. I saw them walking together, loaded with Christmas presents. I pulled into the side of the road, leaned across, wound down the passenger window and shouted out to them: 'Martin! Julia!' Martin recognised me first and looked awkward. Julia walked up to the car and said: 'Hi!' I noticed a café down a side street and suggested we had a quick coffee. She agreed and I parked up.

Strangely, I remember very little else about that meeting, except that I learned they were both primary school teachers and lived in east London. Probably nothing in particular was said, the new relationship was acknowledged, and we promised to keep in touch. But we never really did. I say 'never really did' because I see from the address book that I had at the time that they later moved to Sheffield, and I suppose they both got jobs in education there. So long ago though. Decades went by without any contact.

One day recently, curiosity about them got the better of me. I did a Google search for Martin Jones, Sheffield, and there was someone of that name who was part of a three-member folk and country group. There was a photo of them. And there was Martin strumming his acoustic guitar with his left hand, which he always used to do at get-togethers at college all those years ago.

Then I stumbled across a video clip of the group. They sounded pretty good. They were playing at a folk festival held on the outskirts of Sheffield. Martin's voice, which had always been on the thinnish side, had 'filled out'. He still had that habit of bending forward and playing the guitar as if it was electric: I remembered his wonderful imitation of Marc Bolan. He even had the same hair. Laughter and a sense of the ridiculous had never been far away from Martin and that was one of the reasons I'd liked him.

The group had a Facebook page and on it were more clips of their concerts. One looked as if it had been filmed in a pub. I watched as Martin introduced their next song. He said it had been requested by his daughter and the camera swung away from the group and into the audience where the young woman he'd just referred to was sitting, smiling, pleased at the acknowledgement.

But Martin wasn't the only proud parent caught on camera. Also in view was another older woman, whose distinctive features made me catch my breath. Those high cheek bones and the broad face were unmistakeable. A smile played around her lips, slightly subdued and thoughtful. Perhaps she was exhibiting a deeper joy. This was Julia, more than 40 years on from the last time I'd seen her. I looked and I looked. And a flood of happy memories swept over me.

Here was a woman who had wanted to marry me. Here was a daughter who, if I'd decided or acted differently, could have been mine. Was she their only child? I had it in my mind that they had two, but I don't know where that idea came from.

I tracked down this little film in the dead of night during one of my bouts of insomnia, which was proving to be a growing problem. Strangely, the very un-staged, ordinary quality of the recording added to its poignancy. I had no ticket to their private event. I had gate-crashed a musical evening in a Sheffield pub and was lurking at the back, hidden in the shadows, disturbed by a ghostly daguerreotype of what my life could have become. And ever since my furtive journey into the past, I've been unable to get those smiling faces out of my mind.

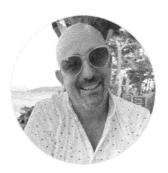

Graham

I NEVER WANTED to settle down in my twenties and well into my thirties. I think maybe I was too careful or had commitment issues. I also wanted to be in the right relationship, which maybe I did have but not necessarily at the right time.

John

I FIND IT hard being around families or men who are fathers. A typical example is with work colleagues. Having to celebrate their pregnancies and showing up with their new-borns can be incredibly hard and you cannot escape. Another example is the many couples who at first were unable to have kids, but somehow managed to have two or three in the end.

Storyhouse, Chester, 10 September 2022

I PLAN TO frame a scrappy sheet of A4 paper on which is scrawled my almost illegible notes. Then I'll hang it on the wall above my desk so that I can remember the most important speech of my life. I made it at the Childless Festival in the Storyhouse Arts Centre, Chester, on 10 September 2022. I joined the men's panel, after being recommended as a possible speaker. I was full of trepidation. I am not used to public speaking and find it so nerve-racking that I have stayed on in jobs longer than I would have liked to just so that I could avoid making a leaving speech. But this was different: I was speaking on a topic that was close to my heart and at last I had a forum in which to express my thoughts. The adrenalin rush carried me through. The audience of about 60 comprised mostly women: they are more usually identified with the issue and feel easier about attending such an event. This was the first men's panel that there had been.

A leading light of the childless movement, the author Jody Day, came up afterwards and said the men's panel had been the most important of the whole event. She added that she found my presentation the most moving of them all. I must have done alright. So, what did I say in my 10-minute address, the most important that I had ever made?

I SHOULDN'T BE here at all. I should be in a pub on Dartmoor with my partner at a family reunion. By not being there I haven't made myself too popular. But I had to be here. There was no way I could miss this event. Quite apart from the fact that the assembled ranks of children and grandchildren would have made me feel pretty dreadful.

I'm a little bit different to the other guys on the panel. I'm childless by circumstance, not because of infertility. So, that's it really. I should perhaps just stop there and hand over to the next speaker. You see, there's nothing to point to. It just didn't happen. This condition − if that's what it is − is harder for the childful (if there isn't such a word, then perhaps there should be) to understand. I was speaking to a married friend of mine about it. He just didn't get it and I had to explain. He thought I wanted to carry on with my bachelor life, galivanting around the world, while idly and thoughtlessly becoming a biological dad without responsibilities. Only after I kept on trying to get him to see that I wanted to be a father *and* assume all the duties of being a father or parent did he cotton on. Men and women who just fall into parenthood invariably find it impossible to understand that the childless can actually yearn for what they have. It is a paradox. But there seems to be a structural incomprehension at play here. A yawning gap of misunderstanding.

To put some flesh on the bones, I need to look back. Back to wrong decisions, bad judgements, an abortion, a miscarriage, a broken engagement. Mistakes. To ex-girlfriends with whom having a child might have worked if I'd stuck at the relationship. Then I must factor in bad luck, complacency and the mantra: I just didn't meet the right person.

You see, men get broody, too. This was particularly so for me in my early forties. I spent about 15 years purposely not having deep relationships because potential partners were too old to become the mother of my child, or were divorced and didn't want any more children. Even though I was compatible with these women to a greater extent than I had been ever before. Thus, I stabbed myself in the back when suitable women turned up because they were unable to help me fulfil my dreams of becoming a father and a parent.

Is it too fanciful to say that my excessive caution did in fact show a heightened sense of responsibility? Choosing not to have children within a less than satisfactory relationship means I avoided pain: my own, my future wife's and my children's. Nor did I bring more children into an overcrowded planet.

So, what about now? I realise that no son of mine will ever phone me up and say: 'Hi, Dad! How are you? Can we go and see Spurs next weekend?' Actually, that would only bring more pain. But what I will hear is: 'You could always adopt, you know' or 'Why don't you get a dog?'. These coping strategies don't interest me. In fact, I despise them and they make me angry. As a writer, I must speak the truth and face it head-on.

Empty is the name of the play I have written about male childlessness. In it I used the two words 'underused' and 'unused'. Because this is the real issue here: being unfulfilled at the deepest level.

In recent months the thinking has shifted from the pain of being fatherless to the pain of being parentless. And this later reincarnation brings with it a realisation that carries far more hurt than the first one did. Being a parent involves nurture at a profound level. It calls on an adult to turn his or her life experience into something rich for the benefit of their offspring. To turn love into an educative tool for children. What's more, I would argue that nurture is an elemental need and, if there is no outlet for it, it can numb that person spiritually. It can also be psychologically dangerous.

If I look back at my career I realise now that these feelings of deprivation were at play when I moved out of journalism and into teaching, where the opportunities for nurture were greater. Strange how the unconscious drives us, the motivation for such action only becoming clear later.

So, what of the future? Emptiness is everywhere. I think of the lack of any legacy and wonder who will be there to look after me in the future.

Jody Day shows in *Living the Life Unexpected* that women can repair the damage of being childless not by choice by putting two fingers up to society's pronatalist tropes and return to their essential selves and lead a fulfilling life. This transformation is bolstered by the stark medical fact of the menopause, after which it is physically impossible for a woman to conceive.

Can men rescue something similar from the wreckage? For some reason it seems more difficult and I'm not sure why. At least, for now. Quite how that escape route can be found evades me. One thing's for sure: society's glib view that men can become fathers into ripe old age is unhelpful. The theory goes that men can procreate until the day they die. True on one level, but in practice, such an event seldom happens. Just look around. You won't see many Mick Jaggers strutting their stuff on our streets.

I am 71 and the pain gets worse, not better. It needn't have been like this.

John

NOT BEING A father is the biggest loss of my life and it makes me feel so sad. The grief is mixed with anger, frustration, unfairness, hopelessness and envy. People generally have absolutely no idea how incredibly tough and heart-breaking being childless is. I have received many hurtful comments over the years and I guess they mostly come out of simply not knowing or understanding.

Alastair

SOCIETY ASSUMES EVERYONE is a parent. They forget many people are not. That really gets up my nose. The grass is not greener on the other side, so stop trying to tell me how lucky I am not to have a child.

Leaving a Legacy

I REMEMBER THE time at school when our Divinity teacher (before the subject was renamed Religious Studies) got the class to read out Genesis Chapter five from the *Bible*. I'd never heard such gobbledygook in all my life.

Verse three says: 'And Adam lived an hundred and thirty years, and begat a son in his own likeness, after his image; and called his name Seth.'

Verse four: 'And the days of Adam after he had begotten Seth were eight hundred years: and he begat sons and daughters.'

Verse six: 'And Seth lived an hundred and five years, and begat Enosh.'

And so on for 30 or so verses. Quite what the teacher was aiming to achieve with this pointless rendition I have no idea. But I was left with visions of a dry and dusty land where men with grizzly beards sowed their wild oats in a never-ending spree of procreation. All very male.

And I couldn't help but be affected by the accumulative effect of the word 'begat' or 'begotten'. What's it mean, sir? To produce children, you stupid boy. Then why don't they say that?

This classroom episode came back to me when I was researching my ancestors. The trip to their old stamping ground – north Oxfordshire – was fun and productive, but once I was back home,

I shifted my attention to ancestry.co.uk to tease out the detail and things turned dark.

Just as with 'begat' in Genesis, the continuous reference to my lot having copious numbers of children furrowed my brows. The 1841 census records that my great-great grandparents, Stephen and Mary, had eight offspring – Thomas aged 15, John 13, Sarah 10, Stephen nine, Henry eight, Samuel five (from whom I'm descended), Daniel three and Eliza one. My great-grandparents, Samuel and Eliza, had four. Some died in infancy, one in the First World War.

But the men, who were either shepherds, agricultural labourers or gardeners, for the most part died intestate with not a penny to their name. Samuel left Eliza £10 in his will, but that was only the value of his effects. They were continually moving from one shabby, rented premises to another. And one – a certain William – spent time in two workhouses, one in Chipping Norton and the other in Whitechapel, London. Each one of them was cripplingly poor.

Yet the children kept on coming. At first, I glibly thought, along with the old cliché, that this happened because they had no electricity or telly to watch, so they went to bed early and made love. In my cultural confusion as a 21st century man, I imagined a scenario in which I saw my forebears leading a carefree existence, producing child after child with a seeming lack of thought. No head-scratching about whether 'in these straitened times' they could afford to have another. Or the extra work that would involve.

I was envious of the way they apparently felt so in tune with the natural processes of life. I allowed myself to hear the laughter and squeals of the children and see their innocent tumbling and running. And nor would I be here today if it hadn't been for my ancestors conceiving Samuel one beery, boozy night in 1836. Lucky devils! They didn't even have to think about the future: little did they know they would be begetting envy decades later.

But I was wrong, of course. Not only did the Nurdens have no access to contraception, they didn't have any sex education or the possibility of having an abortion either. And with the high childhood mortality rate and the need for children to go to work or look after parents in old age, people were forced into having huge families.

Unlike my forebears, I will not be leaving any children behind. This particular branch of the family name stops here. This lack of legacy is an almost universal regret among the childless. Many worry about who will look after them when they are older. Loneliness is another concern.

Michael Hughes, founder of The Childless Men's Community and The Full Stop, admits that he often asks himself: 'Who will come to my funeral? How many people's lives have I touched? What is my mark upon the world?' He has observed, too, that the most valued quality among the men in dramas such as *Game of Thrones* is the possession of a strong bloodline or lineage – and that the less admired characters are invariably childless. This is the unspoken pronatalist trope playing itself out in cultural life.

It's time we defined legacy. A dictionary definition has it thus: 'Legacy is something that is passed on. [It] may be of one's faith, ethics and core values [or it] may be monetary or assets. [It] may come from one's character, reputation and the life one leads – setting an example for others and to guide their futures.'

Here, then, is a source of hope: not having children does not bar someone from leaving an imprint after death. Legacy doesn't have to be a physical entity. It can be merely having a good influence on others that lasts.

Michael Hughes has turned this into a mantra for daily living: 'Make today count', which seems admirable to me. And this is echoed by Sikhumbuzo, another member of the community: 'I prefer living a legacy than leaving one. I have challenged myself to be the legacy.'

I have quoted other childless men here for a reason: I want to show the resourcefulness of this group of men that I have joined. They can find themselves on the margins of society and as a consequence they feel culturally isolated. This, in turn, triggers much painful soul-searching and thoughtful analysis. See how the bleak scenario of a lack of legacy can be turned on its head and become something positive.

One more thought: a legacy may, of course, be negative as well as positive. There is no guarantee that the children parents leave behind – those little Johnnies and Jills, the sons and the daughters – will profit the world in any way. Their influence may be pernicious, however much good nurturing parents do. And that's where the childless, not having any legacy of the offspring variety to focus on, can dictate the terms of their legacy and what they leave to the world. The road ahead, then, is wide and free. In theory, at least.

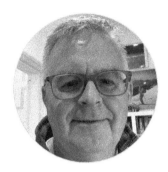

Mike S

NOT LEAVING A legacy and without brothers or cousins with the same surname means the family line will stop with me. That troubles me greatly and, being a keen genealogist, the angst worsens as I grow older.

Ken

EVERY DAY I see I'm just the guy that married her kids' mother. That's all I am in this world. It's heart-breaking. I see the legacy my wife is leaving. Recently her son was looking for a new job. He was telling us about it and I was very interested, asking him questions. I told him to let me know how the interview went. He said: 'Definitely'. He never did. He did call his mother to tell her about it though. Now her grandson's wife is pregnant, so she will become a great-grandmother. I see a legacy growing in my own house, but it's not mine.

The Cute and the Cruel

MEN WHO ARE childless not by choice learn to recognise the warning signs that can get thrown up by certain life events. These triggers of negative feelings invariably emanate from the most normal and common occurrences that have little impact on other people, certainly not a negative one. Some of these are visual, some verbal and others circumstantial.

One of the tropes that frequently crops up is the image of the 'perfect family' seen in public places. So, a trigger can be activated by spotting children playing in the park, particularly if their father is with them. Dad walking his children to school is another that can bring pangs of envy. Quite apart from the never-ending images of the happy nuclear family promoted by advertising; itself an unacknowledged mouthpiece of pronatalism.

Mother's Day and Father's Day are two other public events, albeit ones that are largely recent commercial creations, that can act as triggers. Pretending to be happy when one's partner's children arrive at the house with flowers and presents for their mother can stretch cordiality to its limits. And it can last the whole day and beyond, particularly if they chat about the past and then move onto the present-day and talk about their own kids – and her grandchildren. The polarities are a yawning gulf between the cute and the cruel.

That happened to me recently and the stress of that experience triggered a health event – my blood pressure soared, I had an attack of amnesia and was taken to A&E. The episode lasted several hours. More broadly, this phenomenon undoubtedly has physical manifestations. A common feature of the trigger is a short, dull ache in the chest, which I find can be controlled and eventually dissipated by taking a series of deep breaths.

Father's Day can have similar connotations. I remember going for what I thought would be a quiet walk alone along the river. Except that I kept on meeting families led by a proud father laughing and joking with his sons and daughters on his special day. But, there again, I could have been wrong. Appearances can be deceptive. That father may not have been the biological father and could have been an adoptive parent, a stepfather or a foster carer. And while a family you see in public may look 'perfect' from the outside there can be all sorts of issues going on behind closed doors. The childless man's reactions can be triggered by his own imagination, assumptions and insecurities around parenthood as much as reality. Clearly, someone who is childless not by choice must tread carefully. There are many pitfalls.

Conversations at work is another danger area. All it takes is for colleagues to start chatting about their children and what they did at the weekend and the man who is childless suddenly finds he has an invisible sticking plaster slapped over his mouth. Listening to milestones, achievements and success stories of fertility treatments or high-risk pregnancies is on the list, too, of course. Especially when those happy events have come after years of the couple in question trying to conceive and when one's own experience has been a failure.

It would be wrong to give the idea that when such events are a source of stress for the childless man that he always turns into a mute punchbag of hurt. Don't doubt that there can be a backlash when the pain morphs into anger and even gloating and glee when seemingly happy families experience setbacks. I hate to say this but, hearing about the stresses and downsides of having children, and even the expense, can act as an antidote, too. This is not a pretty business.

One friend of mine says the worst trigger is when you tell a stranger that you don't have children and they respond with: 'You're lucky'. 'Don't they realise anything?' asks my friend.

The range of events that can have this effect is wide and long. Nor is one necessarily safe within the confines of one's family. Just seeing one's nephew going off to college or a niece talking about her first boyfriend can be enough. You can get plunged into the depths just by seeing your own parents spending time with their grandchildren or just talking about them, knowing that you can add nothing to the conversation.

Yet with the pain can also come some relief, even though it is double-edged. As one friend told me: 'Watching my nieces grow up is both lovely and bittersweet.' And he has a kind of cure, ready at his fingertips. 'Movement tends to be a remedy for me, be it walking, running, cycling, as well as being lucky enough to be able to chat to my wife about it.' In the same vein, my partner and I are able to take trips away more or less when we want, something that a family cannot contemplate doing.

These safety routes have to be painstakingly worked out over the months and years. Before that, the childless man (and, of course, the childless woman) will experience countless episodes like those I have listed above. They will experience that familiar dread in the stomach as rooms they are already occupying fill up with arriving families and then reverberate with wall-to-wall family stories. They will wonder why their loved ones never quite seem to get it. But the childless are clever folk and have learned to be ever-resourceful. Some kind of solution is near at hand.

Graham

I'M IN A monthly curry club – four to five blokes meeting up for a curry and a beer. 70 per cent of the conversation is about their family life, kids and all the dramas that go with that. I'm the only one without. I don't think for one minute they consider how I feel. I'm just childless Graham.

Mike S

THE TURNING POINT for me was when attending the 60th birthday party of a close friend. His then mature daughter, whom I had known since she was a child, arrived looking a picture of elegance and my friend was overwhelmed to see her. Suddenly I was completely overcome with jealousy, broke down and had to retire to compose myself. I knew then that I needed help and so sought it with a counsellor. The sessions were very helpful. Obviously, they were not a solution, but they gave me ways of dealing with awkward situations like that.

Last Throws of the Dice

TIME WAS TICKING away. The chances of me becoming a father were fading fast. At times it was too much to bear. Attempts to find a woman in England who wanted the same as me had come to nothing. I had always liked travelling so, without thinking much about it, I decided I needed to be abroad. Below, I describe two episodes in that quest. Looking back, my decision was really just a reckless gamble. I'm not sure I'd do it again.

Lucinda

AT FIRST, I wasn't sure if it was her. She was standing behind a large pillar in the arrivals hall of Cebu airport, her head coyly appearing on one side, then the other, trying to make out if the white man with a sun-reddened face and large suitcase was the man she had come to meet.

I had arranged to visit Lucinda in her native Philippines, having come across her on a dating website a few months earlier. I had been driven to looking abroad for a suitable partner because I had been unable to find anyone in my own country. I don't know the reason for not having struck up a relationship with an English woman who might also want to have a family. Age difference perhaps. I knew I had arrived late at the table, maybe too late.

Lucinda's profile said she was looking for a husband and I just about fell within her preferred age range. She was one of a number I wrote to in the same country. There were some advantages in contacting a woman from the Philippines: she would more than likely speak English and she would have a Christian heritage, which was a positive factor even though I professed myself to be agnostic. Lucinda, in particular, looked lovely in her photos, of which there were many. Unusually tall and slim, with a warm inviting smile, brown eyes and lightly tanned skin. I really did fancy her. Her letters were friendly and avoided being coquettish. And she agreed to me coming over to see her.

Eventually I came face to face with her behind the pillar, her head bowed shyly. I didn't know it at that point, but it was to be the only time that I was to be alone with her. As soon as we shook hands in the dripping heat of the airport, we were surrounded by other people, all older than she was. These turned out to be her family: her mother, two aunts, her brother Tony and various neighbours. There seemed to be no father. Some of them pawed at my shirt, as if to confirm that I had actually arrived. Some were smiling, some were not. Her brother was not.

I was led out of the building to a large van parked outside. I was placed in the middle seat next to her and, once everyone was settled, we set off, with her brother driving. The family lived in Toledo City, on the other side of the island, and it was a three-hour journey across the mountains. Her spoken English was not as good as I had anticipated and I got to wondering if someone had been writing her letters to me on her behalf. I mustn't be too ethnocentric about this I told myself: my Tagalog – her first language – was non-existent.

I tried opening conversations with her, but the noise of the vehicle and her inability to understand and respond made it almost impossible. But I did glean that the family had hired the van and I was expected to pay for it. Luckily, I had some cash. In the end I gave up trying to communicate with her, but I looked across at her from time to time: she was even lovelier in reality than in her photos. I caught Tony eyeing me up suspiciously in the rear-view mirror several times.

On the edge of Toledo City, we stopped and I was told that this was my accommodation. I was glad to see that it was a simple yet decent-looking guest house. I offloaded my case, checked in and got back into the van, all the time following Tony's explicit, arm-waving instructions.

The town spread out along the waterfront, bicycles and tricycles everywhere, jeepneys blaring their horns, cattle being driven along, in and out of the pedestrians. We pulled up at the entrance to what looked like a slum, the structures' corrugated iron roofs glinting in the hot sun. Surely, they didn't live here? They did.

I was led into the narrowest of alleyways running between shacks, the mud at our feet several inches deep. My shoes were filthy with grime within minutes, The walk continued for what seemed ages, weaving in and out of interminable dwellings, each appearing more destitute than the one before. Mothers and children stared at me, the white Westerner, as I walked by. They were curious but they didn't look surprised and I wondered if some of them had been primed that a rich man from England was coming to marry the family beauty.

I had lost all sense of direction by the time we reached their house, which was basic in the extreme. I was ushered in and offered the only comfortable chair, its cushions plumped-up for my arrival. I was also offered tea. Lucinda sat next to me. All I wanted to do was reach over and kiss her. She was stunning, her delicate features a stark contrast to the poverty in which she lived.

Figures loomed at the door to look at the newcomer. Once I counted 12 inquisitive faces peering in at the same time. Giggles and nudges and beckoning of the arms brought others forward. If my mission hadn't had such a serious purpose I would have laughed. All I did was smile nervously. And then there were the glowering features of her brother who never took his eyes off me.

Tony turned on the computer that Lucinda had been using to communicate with me and clicked on a folder. For the first time, he smiled at me, but I didn't warm to his smile: 'You like?' he asked. I noticed that Lucinda was looking perturbed at this turn of events.

On the screen had appeared numerous images of his sister in extremely suggestive poses. I had never seen them before. In one, her short skirt was riding provocatively up her shapely thighs; in another her cleavage was in full view.

'Yes,' I said sheepishly, wondering why I needed to see these posed photographs when the subject was sitting right beside me. Lucinda frowned disapprovingly at her brother as he lasciviously brought up image after image.

My mind raced. Her family was impoverished, yet they had invested in a computer. Conceivably, it was owned by a group of families who, in an attempt to escape poverty, chose some of the more attractive of their womenfolk to advertise online to Western men in need of a young bride. Lucinda's angry glances at Tony suggested that he might be exploiting her looks in this way and she had no say in the matter. There was no doubt that Tony was the head of the family. I even wondered, as I scoured his hard features, whether there might be a connection of a very different kind between brother and sister.

Soon we were on the move again. We retraced our steps back past the huts and out on to the street where the van was parked. We drove to a hypermarket where Tony grabbed a gigantic trolley and, along with the rest of the family, filled it to the brim with groceries. The shopping done, I was pushed to the head of the queue at the till and it was made quite clear that I would be paying. Next stop was the fish market where Tony bought what looked like boat loads. I forked out for it all, of course.

This was turning into a nightmare that I instinctively felt I had to extricate myself from, even if it meant saying goodbye to Lucinda. I knew that Western men in countries such as the Philippines and Thailand were expected to provide for not only the woman but for the whole family. But I hadn't expected it to look like this. If the relationship had started on this financial basis, it was clear that it would continue that way. I was merely a device for lifting the family out of poverty. Any marriage was probably incidental. I would never escape their expectations. I would be a sugar daddy for the rest of my life. The financial outlay I contemplated was horrendous. I regarded myself as a generous person, but not that generous. Provider would be my primary role. It was too awful to contemplate. I had to distance myself from this growing threat. If I stayed I could be trapped. Metaphorically, certainly. But also, given the brooding, sinister character that Tony seemed to be, I could end up being a prisoner in the physical sense, too. Or even worse.

I concocted a plan. If it worked, the end of what was turning into a case of dating incarceration was in sight. I managed to convey to Lucinda that I was feeling exhausted after the journey and wanted to go back to my accommodation to sleep. She told her brother and, much to my surprise, he nodded in agreement. After all, the food I'd bought would last the family several weeks.

They drove me back to the guest house and I said a cheery goodbye: 'See you tomorrow morning.' By now it was dark. Never had I been so pleased to see a set of red tail-lights disappear into the gloom.

I ordered a meal, paid my bill for the night's accommodation and went to bed. I slept fitfully, one ear alert for the noise of a car drawing up and the sound of voices as Lucinda's family came back to check up on me. I had been surprised enough by events as it was. Given the craziness of the situation, anything could happen. But I was left alone.

I tossed and turned in bed. I knew I was letting Lucinda down and I felt guilty about that. I could be condemning her to a lifetime of poverty. But, if I was unwilling to lift her out of that, then better to leave as soon as possible. The truth was that we hardly knew each other and the psychological damage would hopefully be minimal. It may be hard to believe but to quit now rather than later would be easier for both of us. I always project ahead and here I was doing it again. Yes, I felt ashamed of raising her expectations and then changing my mind. I hold my hands up: I was a coward.

I woke to dawn peeping over the plastic curtains. It was 5.30am. I packed my bags immediately and tip-toed down the stairs and out into the street to wait for a rickshaw to pass. I hailed the first one and I was quickly propelled away and dropped at the first bus-stop. Here I could make my way by public transport to Cebu airport and beyond. Which is indeed what happened. I was free.

The next day I received an email from Lucinda: 'Where did you go?' she asked, as she might well have done. 'I wanted to know you.'

'I am sorry. I had to leave. It is difficult to explain,' I wrote. 'I was afraid. I hope you will be happy in your life.'

Magi

WELL, I HAD thought that going to the Philippines represented the last throw of the dice in my desperate quest to become a father. That failed, of course, and that should have been it. I should have accepted my lot. But back in England, after a period of calm, the old hankering returned. I was in my mid-fifties. It was now or never.

Slowly, a plan took shape just as the world of journalism was losing its appeal. Freelancers were being frozen out and sub-editing increasingly resembled stepping on to a treadmill of inconsequentiality. The dice looked at me, winking even, enticing action – and I succumbed.

So, there I was, on the coach to Plovdiv in Bulgaria, my resurrected teaching career beckoning from the horizon of the flat, Thracian plain. I was surging with renewed life and expectation as I had a definite job to go to. I had done my calculations: as a Westerner living in a struggling economy, I would have financial clout not from the salary which I would command (which would be negligible), but from what I would bring with me in terms of accumulated wealth. Age was against me in the dating stakes but personal circumstances were in my favour. Surely, I'd be able to find a suitable woman? Even after the Philippines debacle, here I was taking the self-same route. I felt ashamed, as I had the first time. Even embarrassed and apologetic. Then I reassured myself that life had dealt me a duff hand and I was fully justified in trying to rectify it.

Plovdiv had the most gorgeous girls. And it was the women who seemed to speak the better English and were generally the better communicators. Many of the men looked buttoned-up and contained, not in a self-conscious English way but in a strong, silent way. To smile and laugh was seen as a sign of weakness, sociability a neglected art. To enter a shop was to enter a world of seeming indifference, perhaps a throwback to communist times when entrepreneurship was an unknown concept and sales staff got paid a basic wage, however well or badly they performed. In my worst moments of social isolation, I thought the people grumpy. My over-simplistic analysis was hugely misplaced, of course. I learned later how totalitarianism could impact the whole of a society's psychological aspirations and well-being for years to come.

Most of my students were women, eager to improve their English so that they could land a more senior post in Bulgaria or work abroad in Spain, Britain or the USA. They came to class, dressed to the nines and they seemed to hang on my every word. Again, an example of my vanity and naivety: the arrogance of middle age! Even more surprising since I was not teaching very effectively or imaginatively. Perhaps I was distracted!

I decided to join a dating agency. I guessed that was the way to make contact with those women who were available. In fact, it was called a marriage bureau. Why not cut to the chase? Time was short. Above all else, I had taken myself to Bulgaria to increase my chances of finding a wife and eventually to have children.

So, on the appointed day I went to have an interview with the woman who ran the agency in a poky upstairs room just off the city's main street. She was personable but very direct. 'I have just the woman for you, Robert. She's called Magi and, if you would like me to, I can send her your photo and details. Her English is quite good. Here is her picture.'

I found myself looking at another Plovdiv beauty. She had red hair and piercing green eyes and a look that gave nothing away. She was in her late thirties and was looking for marriage, according to her description. She had a degree in Fine Art from Veliko Tarnovo University, one of the best in the country. She worked as a manager in a factory that made women's underwear.

Magi and I met for a meal a day or two later and all seemed to go well. At least she wanted to see me again. Her English was not as good as the person at the agency had made it out to be, so conversation was challenging. When two people are middle-aged, or edging towards it, one assumes they've lived a lot and have stories to tell. Complexity is the likely order of the day. That needs language and nuance. I wondered – if we carried on seeing each other – whether Magi and I would ever be able to share those difficult thoughts and feelings through language. Of course, my Bulgarian was virtually non-existent and we were in *her* country. But there was no way I could rectify that until I had been there a while.

Magi and I became closer. The winter turned bitterly cold and my apartment, on top of the block just below the uninsulated roof, was freezing most of the time. We developed this giggly routine in which she pretended to be a piece of machinery at her workplace which bobbed up and down a pole, threading cotton. Meanwhile, I held my arms out and her body rubbed against my hands to get warm. We ended up falling about laughing but stayed cold. So, we tumbled into bed where it was only marginally warmer, but nevertheless too cold to take off all our clothes. I don't think I've ever made love with my shirt on before. I went back to England for Christmas and found I missed her.

One weekend in January, when I was back in Bulgaria, she said something which worried me.

She said: 'I am very happy with you now, Robert.'

'Why's that, Magi?'

'Because you are like Bulgarian man.'

'OK. What do you mean exactly?'

'You like watch television.'

My stomach lurched with fear. Had I heard right? 'Just that? Watch TV?' I enquired nervously.

'Yes, you like to be home, relax at weekend, drink beer, do nothing.'

'And that is all you want?'

'Yes, Robert, that is all I want.'

I had been becoming aware that my search for a woman in Bulgaria with whom I could establish a relationship and have children with was involving a number of sacrifices. This was not my country or my language and my love of the arts – particularly in the spoken word – had taken a back seat. It was a situation that I was prepared to tolerate for the sake of the bigger prize.

Magi, despite her degree in art, painted or drew nothing in her spare time. Nor did she have any arty friends. In her job as senior supervisor in a women's garment factory, she was in charge of about 400 workers. It was responsible, gruelling work and in the evenings. she was usually too tired to go out.

Her culinary expectations extended to *banitsa* and *shopska* salad. I went up to her flat one day. Like mine, it was on the top floor of a block. And, like mine, it was freezing cold, the block being devoid of insulation. She slept and ate in just one room. There was one poky window that looked out over smoking chimneys. Untidy pigeons fluttered on dilapidated rooftops. Her bed doubled up as the sofa in the day. And she cooked on one electric ring. She was desperately poor, even as a senior manager in the factory. I was shocked and saddened.

I asked her once in the early days what she did at the weekends. She said she usually drank coffee with the girl in the flat across the landing.

'Do you go out?' I asked.

'No,' she said. 'I cannot. My money is all for rent.'

Here was a woman in her late thirties with a degree but with nothing to show for it. Prior to me she had had a relationship with a Bulgarian man who said he didn't like her large thighs. He wanted slimmer ones. It seems he threatened to leave her unless she had plastic surgery. She acquiesced and had an operation. He was happy with the result but offered no payment and a month later he left her anyway. It was one of the saddest, most pathetic tales I had ever heard.

Everything fell apart after Magi's comment about watching television. I was scared that we'd just drift into a dull, boring existence. I had to be true to myself. I couldn't afford to let her think that this was the extent of my ambitions in a relationship. Perhaps I should have worked at it more, given it a try. But if we managed to rub along satisfactorily now, the differences were bound to come out later. It was another example of me projecting ahead, which had brought my engagement to an end all those years ago. It was all about the avoidance of future pain, what in more confident moments I would call my sense of social responsibility. But really it was just my selfishness and unwillingness to compromise.

Sadly, our relationship stuttered to a hushed halt. I terminated my teaching contract and within a few months I was back in England. Magi and I stopped writing to each other after a few weeks. The experience had left me bereft of hope. I despaired of ever finding a woman with whom I could have kids. It left me more depressed than ever.

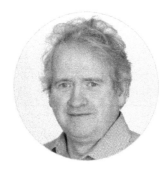

Robin

I THINK THERE are a constellation of circumstances why I didn't become a dad. I was quite shy as a teenager and behind my peers when it came to forming relationships. I was socially awkward. I was behind the pack. I didn't have a deep relationship until my early twenties. In my mid-thirties I was desperate to be a dad: a biological urge and I think a psychological, relational and social need, too. I was aware of being off-track compared to my peers. I didn't fit in with them and I didn't fit with the younger crowd in the pubs and social venues.

Sikhumbuzo

I HAVE BEEN depressed about being childless. Being a father in Zimbabwe is a very important achievement. Failing to have my own child killed my joy.

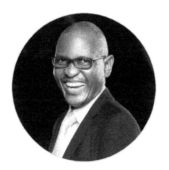

Voices

A LONE VOICE I can handle. I understand it. It's my medium. It speaks of singularity. That's a dynamic I can fathom. I can appreciate its shifts of tone and subtle meanings.

It's multiple voices that disarm me. This morning I walked past an open window of a house further down my street. A myriad voices and cries were pouring out into the damp air. They were using a language different from mine – and I didn't understand a word.

There were children's cries among them. Talking fast. Overlapping. Interrupting. Arguing. Laughing. Unpredictable. Teeming.

And that's what we, the childless, often feel that we miss out on. Life that teems and is unpredictable. Uncontrolled. The disordered life of joy and of passion.

We, the childless, pronatalism's flotsam and jetsam, are often left speaking in hushed tones, leaving us with quietness and regret. Does it have to be like that?

Robin

Cuda, shuda, wuda, dada
There's something missing,
A conversation ended before it began
Scattering thoughts of cuda, shuda, wuda, dada
The latent maelstrom of the none man
There's something missing,
holding a life-wide gap,
breathing wallpaper,
I am whole and incomplete
There's something missing,
first to be left behind,
first to be sent in,
this line is not complete.

Ken

I FEEL DEPRESSED on a daily basis. I never had the joy of seeing my son or daughter born. All the amazing times with them as they grow up. I do know it's not easy, but I do wish I had been a father. There's an emptiness in my heart and soul that will never be filled. I'm part of that minority that isn't seen, heard or recognised. Knowing that the phone will never ring with someone on the other end asking: 'How are you, Dad?' That's heart-breaking to me. Very heart-breaking! It brings me to tears. I know I'll be alone when I get older. That's sad.

Fertile Ground

ON THE DESK in front of me is a tiny, slightly garish, Indian-style pouch made of pink, green and orange silk. If I was to pull it open with my fingers, I would uncover the mysterious object that has remained untouched inside it ever since 2006.

I was given this pocket bag by a south London shamanic healer who I went to see before making a momentous decision in my life. You might recall my Bulgarian story in the last chapter. But what the story didn't say was that before setting out, I paid an expensive visit to this woman who was renowned for her pagan powers. I went specifically to get a steer about whether taking this step at the age of 55 would bring the prize I so desperately craved.

She summoned up my 'male companion spirit' from a cold, northern land. Allegedly. She said that he understood my dream and my predicament and urged me to make the trip as I stood a good chance of finding what I was looking for. In a preliminary conversation over the phone, I had told her why I had booked to see her. In preparation for my session, she had obtained this brightly coloured bag and secreted this object inside. To touch, it felt like plasticine, but it could have been a figurine bought in some junk shop. Was the shape that of a child? I never found out what exactly it was because she warned me not to open it as this would destroy the magic and the powers it possessed. Well, despite my scepticism over the veracity of the enterprise, I resisted opening it, perhaps holding on to a scintilla of hope that this wacky ancient pagan spell might, against all the odds, have something going for it.

Well, I didn't become a father as a result of this south London visit or by living in Bulgaria, so it has to be said that this venture into the esoteric – some would say the world of hocus pocus – didn't work.

I did unexpectedly brush shoulders with pronatalism in the Balkans, but as an onlooker rather than as a participant. I attended the New Year fertility festival of the Survakari, sometimes known as Surva or Kukeri. Its purpose is to drive away dead and evil spirits and to usher in new life and fertility. These rites can be traced back to the wild, religious cult of Dionysus, the god of wine, who was worshipped by the Thracians living in what is now Bulgaria, 1,500 years ago.

Every January the Survakari dancers and mummers, dressed in the most outlandish costumes, go from house to house casting spells and wishing the inhabitants a prosperous New Year. They wear horned animal masks, some in the shape of tall cones, goat costumes and towering feather-decorated headdresses. Round their waists they tie rows of cow and sheep bells which ring hypnotically in rhythm with their dance steps.

The most important of the mummers is the bride and the old man, who may carry a red-painted wooden phallus wrapped in fur. These two characters traditionally enter each house to perform various rituals, which may include a pantomime dance simulating the sex act with the wooden phallus. They generally cajole the young to get together and make love for the purpose of procreation. These are local people who typically may take the whole year to construct their festival outfits, but they never remove them during the event so no one knows who they are. With a few days to go before my return to England, I watched on, feeling numb and excluded.

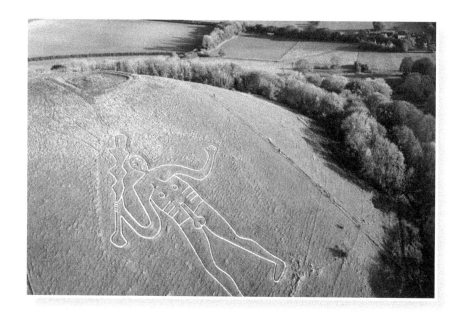

The pagan world of fertility is a lurking, shadowy presence as I write these pages. I'm aware of ghosts and spirits hovering silently over my head. I have so far largely ignored them but now they are crowding in. It is time to acknowledge them and one in particular – the Cerne Abbas Giant. I shall never forget first seeing this naked man carved into the chalk of the Dorset hills. This mysterious 180ft figure, holding a massive club in his right hand and staring out to the west, wielded a frightening power. For a long time, his image has been tunnelling itself into my head.

So, I felt myself being drawn irresistibly back. It was a cold, frost-bound day when I drove, full of wintry expectation, to Dorset. I drew up at the Cerne Giant Viewpoint and got out of the car. I could just make out the Giant's form through the low mist that hung over the hill. Within minutes, miraculously, the mist cleared, moved on by a puff of wind. The mythical beast stood out strong and proud, looking contemptuously down on the tame English countryside. And it was then that I noticed, as if for the first time, his massive erection snaking up the centre of his torso, as far as his navel and beyond. A fertility symbol if ever there was one.

My guidebook told me that no one knew for sure how old he was: he could have been created as early as the Iron Age or as recently as the mid-17th century. Either way, it was a pretty impressive length of time to maintain a stiff. Magic must have been at play, and millions had stood and gazed fascinated on his powerful body. Unknowingly, his makers had dug not just into the chalk, but into the very soul of man.

I watched the mist descend, obliterating the Giant's sculpted shape, and soon he was lost to sight. I abandoned my original aim of getting up close and personal. His presence disarmed me. Shivering slightly, I got back in the car, taking the obscuring curtain as a sign that the pagan drama was over and that my attempted flirtation with this ancient homage to procreation had been brought to an untimely end. I inched out of the car park and drove gingerly back into the 21st century.

There is nothing new under the sun, I told myself as I sat again at my laptop, comforted by the solidity of familiar objects. Procreation has been with us since the beginning of time. In the top drawer to my left lay my mysterious pouch, crying out to be opened. I felt its shape again. It could certainly be the miniature figure of a child, the only one I would ever be able to call my own. But I resisted opening it as I recalled the shaman's words of warning that I should not do so. I was caught in a strange no man's land between believing in its miraculous powers and a rational judgement that it was all a total sham. And that's where I still am today. Unwanted childlessness can take us to strange and dark corners of the mind.

Jan

WHEN MY WIFE and I first started talking about when to have kids (something we both wanted), it was pushed away. My wife became unemployed and changed career. She was afraid being pregnant might affect her chances of finding a good job. When we finally started trying, she was 35 and it just didn't happen. After about a year we sought help and started many rounds of infertility treatment and eventually two rounds of IVF, all without success. She had some minor issues but they should not have prevented her from becoming pregnant, so it was unexplained. Treatments lasted over five years. It was incredibly tough. Coming to the realisation that we would not become parents was absolutely heart-breaking. The whole experience proved to be very hard on our marriage.

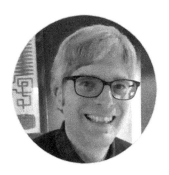

Andy

THE AGONY, THE numbing out, the grief, all this passes, painfully so and slowly. Though they do not pass fully, but remain as touchstones, as scars – I'll never fully heal, but I am living. What is more difficult is the layers I didn't invite in, but barged through as part of society. There was the GP telling my wife and I it is a numbers game. In other words, it would happen with enough sex – the astounding lack of empathy was quite something. On another occasion being told a week is long enough off work to grieve our miscarriage. Yet, for those staff whose child died, they (quite rightly) had as long away from work as required. There was no difference to me, we had both lost a child, but my loss was as invisible as me. I was alone.

Left Behind

BAD TIMING AND bad luck can be reasons for being childless by circumstance. But there may be more complex and subtle factors that those searching for the answer to 'why me?' may need to confront. Dr Robin A Hadley in *How Is a Man Supposed to Be a Man?* writes about how we may need to go back to our childhood to get deeper insights into our unwanted childless state.

I sometimes wonder if my own parents' reticence and shyness over talking about relationships and dating may have contributed to my failure to marry and, consequently, me missing out on being a father. Many people would have seen my parents as Victorian and buttoned-up about matters of sex. For a long time, they were even unable to use the word 'girlfriend' with any ease. And this stayed the same even when I started to have actual girlfriends.

A lack of everyday conversations about emotions, given that they constitute such a central part of life, can skew a child's outlook. It can even induce the feeling that such matters are out of bounds. As a consequence of this, in the end I made my emotional life largely away from the family. For better or worse, I had many partners, which was fun but lacked real meaning because only a disorganised sense of myself was coming to the table.

Even given an unsatisfactory scenario of hands-off parenting, all need not have been lost. Society provides alternative routes, safety nets, rituals and conventions to ease young people into adult life. Strangely, for me, these too went AWOL. Their absence, year after year through growing up, provided a perfect storm of non-engagement.

At the end of secondary school there was no prom or celebration of the fact that studies had been completed or that another stage in coming of age beckoned for me and my classmates. And when, three years later, tertiary education was completed, no one in the family expressed a wish to come to my degree ceremony, so I didn't go either.

18th and 21st birthdays received no special celebration. It was a non-event that went by unrecognised. There were no family gatherings to speak of whereby connections could have been made with relatives of the same age, future meetings planned and so on. There were no, say, barbecue get-togethers or birthday parties. Those ceremonies were eschewed by my parents, mostly by my father. So, later, when I read Edmund Gosse's chilling memoir *Father and Son*, about his experience of growing up in a household dominated by the restrictive practices of the Plymouth Brethren, I identified with much of what he wrote.

In the wrong hands, round-robin letters at Christmas can be ghastly, self-congratulatory things about perfectly functioning children, but at least they serve the purpose of keeping family and friends in touch. Although they received them from other members of the family, my parents never wrote or sent one. It wasn't laziness. It was because they didn't want to trumpet their children's successes, even if they recognised them.

Some of my school friends were clever and successful and their careers reflected that. My father met some of them. My peers were a bright lot who won an unprecedented number of scholarships to Oxbridge. Suffice to say, I was not one of them. In later conversations with his friends, my father invariably spoke of my peers in glowing terms but without a mention of me. I did get my A Levels and my degree but I did not shine so, I presume, I was not worthy of comment in his eyes.

Sport is another catch-all ritual that society provides. Being part of a team can boost confidence and foster a sense of belonging. But with my father it was all about performance. He certainly outshone me academically, but he did at sport, too. I was best at cricket and my ability as a left-handed opening batsman had me picked for my school 1st XI at the age of 16, which meant that, if all went well, I would occupy that spot for the following two summers. But all did not go well: I did not fulfil my promise in any of those three seasons. In other words, I didn't score enough runs. I was dropped from the first team not just in the first of those three but in all three years, which was highly unusual. This gave my father the opportunity to regale others with this anomalous tale, irrespective of the fact that the subject-matter was his own son. Not only that, but to this day I can hear his chuckling at my expense. Fine, but surely it calls for a rider expressing a bit of sympathy for this happening to me. Nothing like this was said.

School theatre productions can also constitute a rite of passage which lifts the curtain on the world for some people. But my reticence and shyness, and a tendency to shrink into the background, meant that I missed out on treading the boards, too. My role in a school production of Gilbert and Sullivan's *HMS Pinafore* was to turn the pages of the score for the piano-playing teacher. But because I couldn't read music, he had to nod his head when he wanted the page turned.

Another coming-of-age trope is independent travel. Looking back on those early years, I now know that what I was doing when I stuck out my thumb on the highways and byways of France, Portugal, Spain and Italy: I was attempting to build an emotional life away from the family. I also hoped that I would meet the love of my life.

Although it took a long time and didn't turn out as I hoped or imagined it would, I did manage to construct a life along the lines that I wanted – and of that I am proud. It just didn't go far enough. In other words, it didn't encompass being a husband or a father. Even when I met wonderful women and established a relationship of sorts with them it never translated into thoughts of marriage because I still had personal 'stuff' to sort out. Somehow, I never felt worthy of their love. Once I did get engaged but broke it off. It would have been a disaster.

I always travelled alone unless I managed to team up with someone else along the way. When it came to flying, I always made my way to the airport under my own steam – in other words I was never taken. And on my return from abroad, I don't remember ever being met. I kidded myself that I was a bit of a loner but in truth I wasn't. Circumstances and unfamiliarity with life-sustaining rituals had conspired to construct a lonesome persona.

Then there are the milestone events of stag dos, weddings, being best man, christenings and funerals, all of which have the potential to pave the way for a young adult towards full membership of society. Again, my involvement in these celebrations was minimal. I have never been to a stag do or been asked to be best man. I probably attended a couple of christenings when I was very young (in addition to my own!).

I've been to very few weddings and have usually felt uncomfortable at them (which probably speaks volumes about my state of childlessness and, dare I say it, my unmarried state). I felt alienated from the ceremony with its strutting, suited males, its loudness and bad jokes that everyone finds funny. I never got the hang of toasts (either I never had a glass to hand or, if I did, it was empty). I could never have made the witty quip from the back of the room that had guests in stitches. I guess I was excessively awkward at social occasions and weddings were the worst of those. It's the imposed conventions of such occasions which turn me over inside. On a brighter note, these days I like the formlessness of parties, as well as holding my own, and I am told that I'm a great host. It's the very lack of convention that makes this possible.

Which brings me to funerals. I understand sadness and melancholy. There is no barrier here. And I have been to a few. At the funeral of my mother, the clearly defined and celebrated figurehead role of the sole grieving son awaited me. But for some reason – perhaps my diffidence, perhaps my sadness – I never fulfilled it. I just stood by and watched as others took over the role of greeter. All very strange. In one way I didn't mind because I could never have performed that trick. I did make a speech about my mother, but it wasn't mainstream. It was idiosyncratic. Not that I intended it to be – I just didn't know the conventions of a funeral address and nobody was there to guide me. Another ritual had gone under the radar. And, of course, I was too off-limits, too ineffectual perhaps, ever to be asked to be a godfather.

Wanting to travel and lead an untrammelled life, I didn't 'settle down', buy a house and get the consequent mortgage until I was 38. Nor did I have much ambition for myself in career terms. I was a competent sub-editor on national newspapers and the normal promotion route is to progress to senior sub-editor and some kind of management role. I eschewed that because I preferred to 'work with the words' and have no responsibility. Thus, another potential route to being a well-regulated, fully rounded, mature adult holding down a senior position went by the way.

There are also particular circumstances which contribute to this feeling of my being left behind. And it's on my brother that I would now like to focus. Tragically, he died suddenly at the age of 23 and it devastated my mother and father – an event they never recovered from.

I was 14 and I was just beginning to grow up through my brother, seeing him rather than my father as a suitable role model on my way to adulthood. One day he was there, the next he was gone, and his shoes have never been filled. I know I would have learned a lot from him over the next five to 10 years. He may have got married and I would have had a template to copy. I certainly would have met his male and female friends, and had the opportunity to mix in interesting circles away from the family. Having that may have acted as a healing balm. I miss him in countless ways.

In addition, not only did I attend a single-sex boarding school from the age of nine until 18, but I soaked up the culture of these alienating institutions in the holidays because my father was a teacher at one as well. A case of the male psyche being divorced from the female mindset twice over. Leading on from that is the notion I have had for decades that my father at heart was a bachelor (he didn't marry until he was 40) who happens, almost by chance, to have married. He embraced the duties of fatherhood with no enthusiasm. In fact, my mother told me that before the birth of his first child he was gripped by fear that he would be unable to be a satisfactory father.

I am aware that the factors contributing to being childless have here become indistinguishable from the factors contributing to being single and unmarried. The latter has, I think, had far more of an influence on the former than I ever realised until I started exploring issues surrounding my childhood. So be it. I seek no sympathy, just some understanding. The double whammy of being left behind comes firstly from the particular parental behaviours I have described and secondly from the fact that I missed out on society's coming-of-age rituals.

But there is no point in sitting gloomily on this. I hope that what I have unearthed may help someone else who finds themselves childless by circumstance reach a kind of understanding as to the reasons behind this sad, unwanted state. Early influences are certainly worth exploring.

Trevor

LOOKING BACK, I suppose I was a bit of a playboy. When I was in my twenties I played the field without a care in the world. I was with some fantastic women but nothing lasted. At first it didn't really worry me. In the end I knew I'd find the right one, get married, and become a father. But it just carried on like that and I found it harder and harder to commit. Now I really regret not trying to settle down with at least two of my girlfriends. So, you stick with what you know best – which is being alone and not expecting anything much. My expectations were too high. Now I'd tell any youngster to work at a relationship, even when it hits the buffers. The trouble was I just expected them to work naturally. I've missed the boat.

The Hidden Perils of Childlessness

WHEN I WAS teaching, sometimes I had a feeling of real satisfaction that a lesson had gone particularly well. The students had been stretched, they had achieved their aims and they departed happy. For a teacher, one can't ask for much more.

I was a TEFL teacher. That is, I taught English to foreign adult students. Most of them were businessmen and women from other countries whose first language was not English. The pressure was on them to learn fast so that they could chair meetings and make presentations in English once they returned to their companies.

On occasions, I found myself taking an inordinate amount of care with their learning. My approach was quite personal and I noticed that this up-close method unsettled some of the older students, schooled in more traditional ways. But they soon realised that there was nothing more to it than my desire to understand their approach to learning so that I could use appropriate methods. I was good at it and I got results. For some of my colleagues, it was a little too touchy-feely, yet it worked.

But, looking at this in a wider perspective, what was I really doing? Were my motives totally altruistic? And why was I successful at it?

After thinking about it, I realised that this was all about nurturing. I was tapping into an elemental drive that most of us possess to some degree. It was, of course, intellectual nurturing, but nurturing nonetheless.

And the reason I was able to draw on this dynamic in the classroom is, I think, because I had never been a father or parent. In my life up to that point I had never nurtured anything except plants in my garden. So, here was another opportunity: helping adults who wanted to improve their English. I had, I suppose, huge reserves of the caring gene. In my keenness to assist them I may have come across as slightly intense, but there you go. Maybe I was lucky to have that outlet. It wasn't the real thing, but it was better than nothing.

But I would like to turn to the question of what happens when those nurturing qualities that good parents usually provide quite naturally are simply not needed. What will be the long-term effect on the childless who have never been able to draw on those attributes?

Qualities that a nurturing parent might exhibit include:
* shared, intelligent decision-making about what's best for one's children
* sensitive care
* sharing with one's partner the joy of being a parent
* providing a helping hand when required
* coming up with creative solutions
* passing on practical skills such as wallpapering and recipes
* exchanging family jokes and stories
* helping with homework
* creating a sense of fun
* playing games
* giving encouragement
* offering guidance, especially when things go wrong
* reading stories
* providing financial security for one's family.

The power of this nurturing drive goes largely unrecognised. More often than not, it kicks in for parents when their child is born.

Mothers and fathers invariably slip effortlessly into the responsibilities of parenthood without even identifying it as a phenomenon. Caring for your own progeny is as natural as breathing. One moment it's just two – a few months later they've turned into a three- or four-person unit. This process in the eyes of those that this privilege has been denied, for whatever reason, can be painful to confront.

Of course, it's more complicated than that. Many parents find they are unable to take on these extra responsibilities with ease and, anyway, the transition to parenthood can take a long time. It is undeniable that some people regret having children. Others can turn out to be poor parents. And mothers can experience post-natal depression, which makes good nurturing a real challenge.

Nevertheless, not being a parent is overwhelmingly seen by the vast majority of our results-driven society as an absence. A sad situation but one that is largely unresolvable (apart from using incomplete substitutes such as fostering or adoption, or even teaching and nursing). And that's that. After all, there's nothing much one can say about the number zero. It all amounts to, well, nothing. Accept it and move on, as they say.

This is bleak stuff and reflects the worst of the despair I felt as I confronted my own childlessness. In writing honestly about all the twists and turns associated with facing up to this painful reality, I lay myself open to the charge that I am causing even more hurt to those members of the childless community who have come out the other side of the tunnel and are navigating the road to acceptance. I'm truly sorry if I've done that.

But I still feel impelled to ask: what happens, at a deeper level, to those men (and women, of course) who never had the chance to be parents when they desperately wanted to be? I am certainly in no position to make authoritative pronouncements that have a universal application. I am no psychologist. All I can do is draw on my own thoughts and feelings about this question and leave it at that.

When confronting this issue, I was scared that my psyche would become 'choked' or 'blocked'. And, at worst, that my mental health would be affected. That it could lead to a feeling of deprivation and the slow, drip-feed of being disconnected from society. There was also a feeling of impotence, of being out of control and there was a sensation of emptiness. I felt I was living a hollow existence and even that my life was a waste. I was worried that further down the line I might turn bitter and resentful. Not only would I never be a father, I told myself, I would never be a grandfather either.

Like many other men and women who found themselves in this dark place, I managed to claw my way back. And that's the story behind the later chapters.

Ken

ABOUT THREE YEARS ago not being a father really hit me, big time. A guy I work with told me his wife was pregnant and that the doctors were a little concerned because of her age: 45. The next day, all of a sudden it hit me like a ton of bricks about never having children. Never being a father. Never holding my new-born. No one to nurture. When my wife and I realised it was never going to happen, I went into deep depression. I was angry. I yelled. I yelled at my wife telling her she or anyone with kids will never understand what it's like. Ever since then every day has been a struggle. I see reminders, triggers every day in real life situations: at work, going to the store, on TV, everywhere. I never will have kids. Oh, just to add, the guy from work and his wife had the baby with no issues or problems. Good for them.

The Fatal Position

'YOUR LEFT ARM doesn't look quite right. Could you do something else with it?' A strange demand. But, there again, I was lying naked on a mattress in the chilly studio of a Brighton photographer I'd met only half an hour before. Flexibility was the name of the game.

Had I taken male martyrdom too far? Was my decision to be part of this project, which was designed to highlight the issue of male childlessness, a case of misplaced altruism? Time would tell. Anyway, for now I went along with it. I followed the instructions I'd been given and changed the angle of my left arm. I was told that was better. The shooting started.

I suppose there was also an element of defiance in choosing to contribute to this photographic essay about childless men. I wanted to prove that these days men are not afraid to show their vulnerable side. Besides, very few of my brothers had volunteered, so I somehow felt duty-bound to. The scheme, funded by the Arts Council, was entitled *Dad's Not the Word* and followed on from the first project which was about non-mothers – called, of course, *Mum's Not the Word*.

I had taken the train to Brighton to meet the award-winning photographer, Denise Felkin, in her studio. As I stepped onto the train at Clapham Junction, childbirth – or its absence – couldn't have been further from my mind. But, as we sped through the Sussex countryside, the import of what I was about to do came home to me. I would have to take all my clothes off, lie in the foetal position and then be photographed, as Denise had explained in her heads-up, honest email. I shrugged off my mild fears. It was an artistic decision. It would be fine.

Denise and I touched elbows, Covid-style. She led me up two flights of stairs to her tiny studio in which an array of massive, light-reflecting sheets hung from the ceiling. In the centre of the floor was a double mattress. Suspended above it was a gantry to which was attached a camera, its lens pointing downwards, accusingly.

She showed me examples of her work from *Mum's Not the Word*, to which the *Independent* and the *Guardian* had devoted features. There were the bare bodies, lying on their side, of at least 10 childless women. Enough of their faces was visible for them to be identifiable. They looked beautiful, the rhythmic repetition of their identical postures creating a sad but stunning spectacle of loss and grief. I felt proud to be taking part in the male version.

Denise had asked me to bring my own duvet cover which we laid over the mattress. She said that she would be operating the camera from her laptop. She asked me to lie on my side, fully clothed: literally, a dress rehearsal then. She would be asking me to change the position of my arms from time to time in order to achieve the most natural-looking posture.

She set up the camera, adjusted the lighting and smoothed out the duvet cover. The problem was that, on this September morning, the sun kept going behind clouds. This forced Denise to change the angle of the reflectors to compensate for the lack of direct sunlight.

She was all set. 'Right, when you're ready we can move to the next stage.' Which was the cue for me to go behind the screen and strip off. I reappeared and lay down. A few more adjustments to the camera equipment.

'Could you move your left arm a little nearer to your face, almost touching? Thank you. And I just need to check nothing is visible between your legs, otherwise we won't be able to publish anything.

Okay, checked that. That's fine. I shall say: "Ready" and that'll be the sign that I'm about to take a shot,' Denise said.

There was a long horizontal mirror propped against the far wall, so I could see myself reflected and her behind me examining the image on the computer screen.

'Ready.' There was a click above my head. Then another and another.

'You still don't look very relaxed. Could you do something else with your right arm?' I placed my right hand on my right thigh. It felt more natural than having it splayed across the duvet in what seemed an awkward, horizontal position. 'That's it. Brilliant,' Denise exclaimed. The clicks resumed. This time there were lots of them. I relaxed and at one stage, against a background of sounds from the keyboard and the camera, I felt myself dropping off. I'd been told to close my eyes, so falling asleep was simply the next, easy step to take.

In a series of previous email exchanges with Denise, I had raised the issue of anonymity. She'd told me that I wouldn't have to do anything that I was unhappy about, which was reassuring. What's more, I would be able to approve the final image. In other words, I had joint control. But that wasn't quite the same thing as remaining anonymous.

I asked if she could take some shots of me with my face half-hidden, turned in towards the bed, so that I couldn't be recognised. In the gallery of women's photos, there was one in which it was impossible to know who it was, so there was a precedent.

To my surprise, she liked the results. 'Good. I think we've got it,' Denise said. I put my clothes back on and we looked at the images on her computer. We picked a couple and she printed them out. The printer chugged and spluttered before spewing out the photographs.

There I was, sprawled out on the blue duvet with its silver moons and stars. I was shocked by the size of my stomach, already too large but exaggerated by the foetal-type posture. I looked gross. More to the point, even in those supposedly anonymous shots, I was still easily recognisable. I said nothing, but I am sure she realised from my silence and body language that all was not well.

She produced a piece of paper for me to sign. It was the model release form. As she ran through the different kinds of media that my agreement would allow her to approach, I realised that the range was wider than I had anticipated. I had thought the initiative would amount to an exhibition in a public space and maybe a feature in one of the broadsheet papers. But I was signing approval of my ghastly image to appear on social media. Not just once, but for ever. However, afraid that I would appear wimpish if I objected, I signed the form.

As agreed, she gave me a copy of the photo to take home. I looked and looked at it. I had a sick feeling in my stomach. Any idealistic, or even altruistic, notions about publicising the little recognised issue of male childlessness went out of the window. Self-protection was my only thought. I realised that I had made a monumental mistake in agreeing to take part. Besides, I was a writer and journalist who, in years to come, could be identified in these images by potential editors or publishers. I couldn't take the risk.

Denise said nothing, so I had to. 'Sorry, Denise, I can't let this image out into the wide world. I'm sorry. I've made a mistake.'

She looked disappointed, not surprisingly. But, in response and to her credit, she took the form and fed it into the shredder. Relieved, I watched it being torn to tiny pieces.

'Don't worry,' she said. 'I know this can be a very emotional situation for people. When I photographed a woman for the first project, she was so upset she spent the first half-an-hour in tears. I must, however, send the digital image to the Arts Council to show how I've used their grant, but I will not use your photo in any other place.'

I'm sorry I've wasted your time,' I muttered. She shrugged her shoulders. I slinked out with a mixture of relief and guilt. The journey back to London seemed longer than the one coming down.

A few weeks later Denise wrote, attaching her completed digital booklet, *Dad's Not the Word*. I looked at the images of the other men lying in the foetal position, about 12 of them in all. Despite their undeniably intrusive quality – the faces were all recognisable – there was a dignity and brazen honesty about them that I admired and even envied.

At the back of the book, Denise had faithfully reproduced my words. But where my portrait should have been, she had placed an empty, black oval. That eerie egg-shape was a stark symbol of my vacillation. It was also a potent symbol for everyone childless not by choice. What's more, I told myself, I had failed in my aim of showing the world that men were no longer afraid of revealing their vulnerable side.

John

THERE IS NOTHING more important than putting a child into this world, a small being to pour all your love into. It's not just women who can feel like that.

Trevor

I HAVE FELT broody in the past and sometimes I still do, although I know it's almost definitely too late now. Besides, with all the dangers around late fatherhood, I wouldn't want to take the risk. It's so frustrating because I know it would have been possible if I'd taken different decisions. As a man, I've missed out on one of life's great events: being a father.

In Praise of Complexity

I'VE OFTEN THOUGHT that the criticism non-believers level at people of faith is unfair. With nothing to lose, because they literally have nothing to lose, they are free to pick off their victims at will, accusing them of hypocrisy, double standards, sanctimoniousness and so on. Having a belief in something you cannot see is such an easy target. And I say this as an agnostic myself.

But these rationalists, unswayed by sentiment in their judgement of people, can't have it both ways. If, in their humanistic unbelief, they favour right, good behaviour and respect towards others, they must acknowledge it wherever it crops up. To them, its provenance should matter not a jot because the impact of what happens in real time should be their only yardstick. Right action is right action whatever its cause.

Yet the resulting failure to attest that many good acts do in fact emanate from people of faith – driven by I know not what but by something – is deeply discriminatory. It's as if the rationalists cannot entertain the notion that people so foolhardy as to believe in a deity can nevertheless perform acts of goodness, inspired directly by a belief in that deity. It suggests that their own philosophical system is as flimsy and uncertain as that of the believers.

More than that, I would contend – again, I repeat as an agnostic – that more and deeper acts of goodness come from believers than non-believers. Perhaps non-believers are expending so much energy on shoring up the rickety structures of their own rationalism against the strong evidence of an antithetical spiritual dimension that they have no room left for any fresh, sympathetic assessment of otherness.

These thoughts came to me as I reflected on a gathering that my partner and I had just attended at the Methodist Central Hall, Westminster, London, one November Sunday afternoon. The title of the service was 'Saying Goodbye'. The occasion was one of a series of remembrance events for people who had 'lost a child at any stage of pregnancy, at birth or in infancy, whether the loss be recent or 80 years ago', as the publicity material of the organising charity, the Mariposa Trust, had it. 'In addition,' it went on, 'anyone who has been through fertility treatment or who has never been able to have children for whatever reason, is most welcome.'

It was an event that we were inevitably drawn to in our several ways. Mariposa, a secular charity, regularly holds these services, presided over by a Christian minister, in cathedrals in Britain and occasionally in other countries. 'We think that a cathedral setting lends the meeting a sense of occasion,' said a representative. Holding a Saying Goodbye service outside of a cathedral setting was unusual but the content is the same, whatever the venue.

There was another reason why I wanted to attend the Methodist Central Hall. My activist grandfather, Stanley James, had made a public speech in the self-same arena a little over 100 years previously. On 9 March 1920, he had spoken on the subject 'The Rebirth of Christianity'. It was a lecture in the *Crusader* series, the eponymous magazine which he edited.

As we listened on that cold winter's day to the sad stories of baby loss and families' attempts to come to terms with that tragedy, I was also picturing my maverick grandfather standing on that stage addressing the audience. And I realised the irony of the situation: Stanley had seven children, my mother being number five. And there was I, a century later, childless, wondering why.

The hall was full of lights – Christmas tree lights, purple lights playing around the backdrop of the massive organ pipes and, most importantly of all, a few hundred tealights. These were on three trestle tables at the front of the stage, each one representing a baby which had died – or for the childless, a wanted baby who had never been born. Participants were asked to add to the existing displays by marking the memory of their lost child. We walked to another table to the side on which were a number of unlit tealights. My partner lit one for her son who died as an adult from a heart condition. I lit a candle for my never-to-be child. We walked back to our seats hand in hand. There were tears. Back in my seat, I looked up and saw another illumination: a garish green display spelling out the word 'Exit' above a locked door.

People read poems, sang songs, offered up prayers. At the end, members of the charity came to speak to us. They were caring, some were Christians, some were not. The compassion of that event was beyond reproach. A rationalist, feeling threatened perhaps, might have searched within the format for an opportunity to be disputatious. Maybe they would criticise the unthinking sentimentality; or the lack of awareness among those participants who failed to see that their baby's death had been caused by cuts to the health budget; or any number of disparities. Yet, encumbered by an obsession for over-intellectualisation, they probably would not have cared as those people cared. There's only so much that the human soul can do. It just depends where you decide to put your energies.

One more thing: grief experienced on such a scale has about it a quality that has much in common with the jumble of thoughts and feelings associated with faith, in which we may hear Wordsworth's 'still, sad music of humanity'. Or understand Hamlet when he said: 'There are more things in heaven and earth, Horatio, than are dreamt of in your philosophy.' A truly lived and committed life is chaotic, full of contradiction, uncertainty and complexity. I speak, of course, as an agnostic.

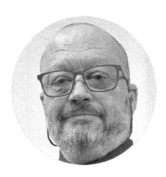

Russ

I STILL FEEL THE discomfort but the breakthrough came when I took 'being a father' out of my identity. It was similar to the way I approach other things in my life. I try to focus on my skill and things which make me happy. I write poetry, I help others, I rescue animals, I ride a motorbike. Conversely, I am not great at sports or playing an instrument … Not being able to be a father is not something I have failed at; it is something that I was never meant to do.

Sikhumbuzo

MY WORK HAS loss reminders. As a pastor, I must christen children. And I write Christian songs for children. Each time I do, my grief is activated.

Back to School

I WAITED FOR the headmaster in the very same room in which I had my first ever lesson as a four-year-old. I remember that September day vividly, 66 years ago. Miss Brown, a tall, large woman wearing a long, black Mother Hubbard dress was our teacher. I was frightened of her as she towered over us.

There was the smell of wet clothes that September morning in 1955. And the grassy whiff of the straw hats that the girls wore and the pungent aroma of hot, displaced bodies that wafted from the pile of ancient mats stacked in the corner. Those mats were used for our after-lunch rest when we were supposed to close our eyes and sleep. There were two types – rush ones made of natural fibre and the canvas ones that looked like pieces of rejected tent material. At rest time, as the class jostled each other to grab the mat of their choice, I always hoped (I always hung back from the heaving throng) that there would be a rush one left for me. It didn't always work out like that because there were fewer of those, so I often had to make do with a canvas one.

That first day seemed to go on forever. I remember the big wooden letters of the alphabet, painted in different colours, that we had to draw round in order to create the shape on paper. We were given plastic cups to drink our fruit juice from at break time. Some

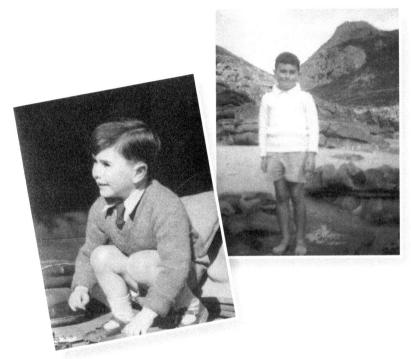

of the children cried, missing their mothers. I missed my mother too and couldn't wait to get home, but I didn't cry.

As I waited in that room replete with history all those years later, the secretary brought me a cappuccino in a special mug which had the school's crest on it – a memento of my visit. Why had I asked my old junior school to let me through the gates for a walk down memory lane? I'm not sure. But, as with so much in this enterprise, I was following a gut instinct. If I didn't do it now, I never would. Perhaps I needed to taste life when it was innocent, before the knowledge of adulthood kicked in.

The memories came flooding back. The school had expanded so there had, of course, been additions to the buildings – walls knocked down and other walls erected. It is odd how one feels affronted about such events, as if one had rightful ownership of the infrastructure. I realised that they were right about smells – that they are some of the most vivid sensations of one's youth. The lunch had been brought in stacked wooden trays in the back of a van from a Hertford company called Bridens. Fridays were potentially special days when it was fish and chips, a meal we never had at home. So, there was some cachet, something illicitly adult, about eating fish and chips, quite apart from the taste itself. As we sat in class on Friday mornings, we waited for the sound of the van drawing up, then sniffed the air. Disappointment ran through my classmates if we detected soggy cabbage and an absence of cod. But when we got what we wanted everyone had a spring in their step. I also remember, a while later, when Friday fish and chips stopped altogether. We never knew why.

When I was about seven, I went up to Miss Taylor's class. We all loved Tay, as we knew her, because she was so kind and understanding, and never became angry. She gave me an encouraging diet of red stars for my maths sums, occasionally even a gold one. She was small, dark and quite glamorous, which I think means that she wore red lipstick, but I couldn't be sure. In the fringe of her otherwise black hair, she sported a white streak. Was it a natural idiosyncrasy or had she dyed it for effect, I wondered. Of course, I never found out.

I wish I still possessed some of those exercise books containing my shining red stars. But what I do have are the termly reports, stapled together between the covers of a drab, dun-coloured book. They range from summer 1958 to summer 1960; seven terms. There were no reports for the first nine terms. I suppose because there is a limit to the number of intelligent comments that a teacher can make about a child's construction of plasticine figures.

I wasn't the best in the form, but I was one of the best. It's all so simple, really. If I hadn't warmed to Tay, I wouldn't have done as well as I did. She gave me a quiet confidence. She understood different pupils' learning styles.

Nevertheless, my recollection is that I always felt quite tense in class and produced only mediocre work. But these reports show that I was pretty good. Summer 1958: 'A very good first term in a new form. Robert is a bright boy and works well. Conduct: Excellent. A most pleasant boy.'

Easter 1959. 'Arithmetic: A very pleasing term indeed. Robert's output has increased enormously. He is very accurate. Mental Arithmetic and Tables good. Conduct: A delightful pupil in every way.

Summer 1959: 'Robert has worked very well this term. He shows great promise in all subjects. He works well on his own and is well able to organise others.' Well, that last comment came as a surprise. 'Conduct: Excellent. Robert is a lively, likeable boy.'

Easter 1960: 'Robert has had a rather disappointing term. He gives the impression that if he showed more energy and determination he could produce good work, but at present he tends to do rather less written work than most others in his age group, and what he writes is often a little 'young' in content.' Those comments concur more closely with my adult memory of those interminable, cold, frosty winter days, aged eight.

I seemed to have bounced back in my last term. Summer 1960: 'Robert has had a very good term and worked extremely well. Writing and general appearance of work has improved. Robert's English and Arithmetic are both very good and Robert's difficulty with Arithmetical problems would be overcome if he would "sit and think"!' I came fourth out of 25 in the class, and in the exam scored 86 per cent in English with an average across subjects of 77 per cent.

Tay could play the piano, too. And every morning at assembly, the hymn books were handed out and we sang the one she'd picked for that day. One of her favourites was 'Eternal Father, Strong to Save', with the equally memorable line: 'For those in peril on the sea'. We sang that on days when the weather was a bit stormy.

But her all-time favourite contained the lines: 'There is a green hill far away, Without a city wall.' I genuinely asked myself over and over again why she liked it so much when it seemed rather a sad city – it didn't have a city wall when it really should have had one. Only years later my mother explained the syntax. It *did* have a city wall. 'Without' here meant 'outside'. Language can be so confusing.

The following year we had our lessons down the road in the Garden House. We felt quite special marching off from the rest of the school to our spacious classroom in this calm and peaceful property on the edge of Bengeo. Out of the back window we could see the church clock and during particularly boring lessons we watched the slow progress of the minute hand as it inched towards lunchtime.

Strange what one remembers. One day as we walked in crocodile pairs along the pavement to our class, we heard an almighty explosion. It came from the sky and on looking up we saw a strange plane with a double tail and a square empty space towards the rear end. I later learned (well, a few minutes ago after consulting Google) that it had what is known as a 'twin-boom tail'. It might well have been a Hawker Siddeley Vixen, which was in operation at that time. That plane was built and tested by the Havilland Aircraft Company which was based in nearby Hatfield, so the evidence is strong. What we had heard was the breaking of the sound barrier, the grown-up world obtruding in a dramatic way.

I had a crush on a beautiful, shy, brunette girl in my class. I am ashamed to say I cannot remember her name. I was smitten and tongue-tied in her presence. One day in art class she was drawing a house. Not one with just a red central door, two windows to the side and three upstairs. Oh no! This was a far more complex and aesthetically satisfying design. Where her walls, made out of authentic yellow Hertfordshire brick, met the roof she had introduced a crenellated effect. I was sitting next to her, spellbound by her work. Suddenly a big boy called Richard turned round to look at what she was doing. He had a large pink face and was good at sport. He grabbed her picture and mocked it for its unnecessary artistry. 'Walls and roofs are not like that,' he bellowed in her ear.

I leapt to her defence and rejoindered that if she wanted to draw her walls like that she was perfectly entitled to do so. 'Besides, they look jolly nice,' I added.

The teacher – Mrs Wilson I think it was – introduced a rota system for walking back to the main school. Each day a different pupil was top of the list and could pick who to walk with at the head of the line. I dreaded my turn coming because all I wanted was to walk with my beautiful girl but knew that I was likely to be too shy to go ahead with choosing her. Indeed, that is what usually happened. On the few occasions when I did choose her, I could never think of anything to say. But my classmates were observant and knew that I loved her. My blushes probably gave me away. So, when I chose a boy from my class instead, they jeered a little and asked: 'What about her, then?'

When it came to the Nativity play in December, I was chosen to play Joseph. Who played Mary? She did, of course. Had the kindly Mrs Wilson arranged it? I don't know but, luckily, I had nothing to say so the part was perfect. And I got to stand near her in a patriarchal manner. There is only one thing to add to this romantic tale: where is she now?

I had a teacher whom I didn't like. She clearly didn't want to be there. I remember one day she told us about her husband's work. She described some enormous machine that he spent all day working on and I realised later that it must have been an early computer. We were meant to be impressed but I don't think we were.

My mother used to drive three of us to school. Right at the end of the journey, there was a tricky right turn at the top of a hill, so some challenging clutch and brake co-ordination was required as traffic invariably hurtled down the hill in the other direction. One frosty February morning, our car glanced another and the headlight was smashed. We grabbed our satchels and were ushered away to school, leaving my mother to exchange addresses with the other driver. It was a disruption to our daily ritual, and it unsettled me.

There was a boy we nicknamed Wyatt Earp, but I don't remember why. And there was a boy with white fuzzy hair called Jasper Gripper who was tough and good at football. With a name like that I guess you have to be athletic.

We played football in the Dell, a deep depression of land surrounded by trees. It was a tiny pitch, so lots of goals were scored, some even by me. But most were solo efforts by a little fair-haired boy called Johnny who was a wizard dribbler. I wonder if he ever made it at senior level.

But what I did see on my return trip as I scoured the boards for names of past pupils was a complete surprise. That name was Oliver Skipp, who, as I write this towards the back end of 2021, is a promising first team player for the club I support – Tottenham Hotspur. When I left the school in 1960, Spurs were about to enter their wonderful double season. That December my father took me to my first match, which we won five – two. Seeing Skippy's name gave my research a satisfying circularity.

Football, school reports, red stars, mental arithmetic, hymns, rush mats, the smell of fish and chips and puppy love: the artefacts of hope and expectation, the building blocks of manhood, the designs of dreams. So, just why did these harbingers of hope never get beyond the drawing board?

Chris

I HATED BOARDING school and I think it's to blame for me never having children. I was cut off from the family I loved for months on end and I think I turned into two people. On holiday I was one person (mostly happy), and at school I was somebody else (mostly lost). I coped with school but that was all it was. Coping. I wasn't happy. So, when it came to meeting girls, I felt inadequate and awkward, and I never really recovered from that. I was married but we split up after five years, so that was that as far as family was concerned.

Think Yourself Lucky
You're Not a Dad, Mate

I WAS HAVING a drink with my mate, Tony, the other day. He's married to June and they've got three kids, so he doesn't get out much. It was good to meet up for a pint – it'd been a while.

'I don't know why you keep going on about missing out on being a father,' he said, looking at me over the top of his glass. 'You don't know how lucky you are.'

He asked me the last time I hadn't slept all night because the baby was crying. When I had felt so knackered that I could hardly drag myself to the kitchen to make a cup of tea. And when was the last time I spent half an hour getting ready before jumping in the car to drive off somewhere. I had to admit that those scenarios were not a common part of my life.

'I bet your house doesn't constantly smell of pee,' he went on. 'And I bet it's quiet most of the time. And that you're free to choose when you want to be alone. I never get that – the kids always come first.

'This is the first evening I've had out in months. Never have enough money either. We're always having to buy new clothes for the kids, games, phones, football kit, you name it. The oldest one will be at university before you know it. More expense. Let alone coping with all the worry about exams, drugs and girlfriends.'

Tony said he never felt relaxed these days. There was always something to worry about. He'd been passed over for promotion at work, he said, because he'd lost his edge, which he put down to constant fatigue. 'And you say you want to be a father?' he concluded. I looked down at my pint and said nothing. I almost felt ashamed at the selfishness of my single state.

We changed the subject and by the end of the evening Tony had recovered his sense of humour. But, when I was alone again, I reflected of the advantages of remaining parentless. I also did some research. In the 2023 Fertility Report on the Legacy website, I found that an older father runs the risk of producing a child with potential issues – autism, Down's syndrome, a greater tendency to bipolarity and reduced fertility, as well as a possible low IQ. In addition, Legacy reports that in a survey of men, 70 per cent overestimated the age at which male fertility decline began or didn't know male fertility declined at all. Once I'd opened the gates, a tsunami of further objections came flooding in.

Then I recalled a recent family gathering I'd been to. There had been four siblings in attendance, three of whom were divorced, one of them twice. In addition, there had been two marital separations, one son not talking to his father and another cut off and hardly ever meeting. The UK divorce rate currently stands at 42 per cent. If there are children involved, and there usually are, then the consequent hurt and blame is made infinitely worse.

Even within marriages that do last there can be deep problems: absent parents, alcoholic parents, drug-dependent parents, abusive parents and, well, just not very good parents. I say parents but the problem overwhelmingly lies with fathers.

It's not guaranteed of course that remaining childless allows one to escape all the problems of marriage and parenthood – stepchildren often see to that – but it definitely reduces the chances. Don't these observations go some way towards convincing the involuntarily childless that their lot is not quite as bad as they thought it was?

The more I delved into the issue, the more I realised it was a tangled web. And, interestingly, the ethical dimension increasingly came to the fore. At the risk of sounding like some guardian of the nation's morals, I would like to create a link between being reckless, or at least thoughtless, and being the cause of pain. When people rush into a marriage, maybe impelled by infatuation or the fear of being alone, they are running the risk that that relationship may one day come to an end.

Childlessness is universally seen as an absence. But dig a little deeper into the reasons for being childless by circumstance and one may unearth some rather interesting things. For example, the man who finds himself in this position may be there not because of, say, bad luck, but because he has an unusually developed sense of social responsibility.

Decades ago, I was engaged to be married but I called it off because I knew I didn't love my fiancée enough. It may have worked for a few years but, in the end, I probably would have met someone else and so would she. Or the relationship may simply have ground to a halt. By then we might have had children and their pain would have been added to our pain. I foresaw this possibility and held back. I might argue that that amounts to being prescient and wise. Self-sacrificial even. Maybe excessively so, but there it is. Oh yes, and I've since heard that she is now happily married with kids.

Perhaps all this sounds weird. But what about those three failed marriages and the estrangement from their sons that I mentioned before? When will they ever get challenged for the hurt that their lack of responsibility has caused? Given the level of pain that has been a feature of those failed relationships, why should they not be asked to justify their life decisions, just as childless men later in life are asked to justify their desire to be an older dad?

People are reluctant – too cowardly even – to explore divorce and separation as deeply damaging states, not least for the children involved. There seems to be a taboo about making such a challenge.

Society lets the statement 'the children have accepted it' serve as a get-out clause for separating parents. The damage is hidden. This reluctance to criticise a failed marriage is just another way in which parenthood is revered. The family rules OK.

But, by remaining childless, it is possible to avoid this potential pain and do society a favour into the bargain. Away from the anger and hurt of not being a parent, there are two quiet, yet powerful, phrases that might help the childless see their situation in a more positive light. One of them could be called 'admirably cautious', the other 'socially responsible'.

Mike C

THE ONLY TIME I find things awkward is when strangers ask the question. It is such a small-talk staple, people talk about their kids and then ask you if you have any. I don't give a shit about being able to say no, but I always feel really bad for the person asking the question, because there's nowhere else they can go with it. It is the small-talk cul-de-sac, the road of no return. But you can't make a joke of it – ha, ha, I ate them, ha, ha. They can't ask you 'Why not?' because you've only just met. All they can do is say 'Oh'. They can't even say 'Never mind' because that would be inappropriate. There is literally nothing they can say that won't have them facepalming later. When I was younger, they might say: 'Well, maybe one day'. But now that I'm 58, there is just a panicky look on their face and a desperate desire to be anywhere else. I have practised in my head things I could say to them that wouldn't leave them hanging in awkward silence, but have never come up with anything.

The Babies Next Door

MY HOUSE KEYS jangled and the baby in the pram looked up. One-year-old Ralph – for once I remembered the name my neighbours had given him – turned his little head and the tiniest of smiles played at the corners of his mouth.

At least I think it was Ralph and not Eva, who was his twin sister. At first, I couldn't tell the difference but, 12 months into their little lives, I thought I had it pinned down. Besides, Eva was the one who was usually asleep, so the chances are it was Ralph.

Their mother is Ukrainian and the father is Lithuanian, and within weeks of their birth they'd asked us to act as a witness for the twins' passport applications. It was from that point on that we got to know them – the wrapping up of the babies before they were put in their double pram and given their 'walk' down our road became a daily ritual.

The wife's mother lived with the family and we could hear her through the wall singing to the children. It was a reassuring sound, the well-practised Ukrainian folk songs being hauled out of her maternal memory. Usually, I'm very sensitive to intrusive sound and it can upset me. But this was joyous and I even looked forward to it. It added another dimension to our quiet, retired lives.

I jangled the keys again, trying to establish a rhythm this time, copying the grandmother's technique. Ralph smiled and now I could see it was a clear smile, a happy one. Mother and grandmother turned to me, and the mother said across the low fence: 'Hello, Rob. How are you today? How's your wife's foot? Is it getting better?' My partner and I weren't married but I let it run. I told them it was slowly improving.

A few weeks before, we had got into discussion with them about soup and how we loved to make our own. 'Me, too,' said the mother.

'Rob makes the most amazing spicy parsnip soup. You must come round and have some with us.'

I couldn't be sure but I reckoned it was the kind of over-the-fence conversation that neighbours used to have before people changed and did their chatting on mobile phones. For years I – and then both of us after we moved in together – had just nodded to my neighbours when we met, hardly managing a word. Before the babies arrived, we used to hear heated discussions, rows perhaps, through the wall and we decided not to be in a hurry to become more friendly with them.

Then Ralph and Eva arrived, and the shouting stopped. And it wasn't replaced by crying; at least we didn't hear it from our side. My partner's maternal instincts kicked in and bonds were quickly made. She knew what to say. 'Eva takes after you, doesn't she?' With the genius of motherhood, she just came out with it. There was no way she couldn't have uttered that immortal mantra. It was an arrow of compassion shot directly at the mother's heart, at the lodestar which is conception, something which has been spoken ever since babies were born. It was totally unoriginal and all the stronger for that. The freshness of new, surprising thinking would have been inappropriate. It marked a gathering in of shared, ritualised caring and living.

After we helped them obtain British passports for the babies, as a token of their thanks, they gave us some flowers, chocolates and a bottle of Lithuanian liqueur.

Just six months later the English couple living on the other side of us had a baby too. She almost had the same name – Evie rather than Eva. The other day we met the father with the pram, taking his weekend paternal duties seriously. My partner pointed out how pretty Evie was. Like the father, she said. I couldn't tell, her eyes so bundled up in fleshy skin. She lay spread-eagled, looking up at the world without blinking. Her podgy, pink arms were at right angles to her body almost touching the sides of the pram. Then her arms flailed in unison as if she wanted to fly. Then, for some unfathomable reason, a line from that wonderful Ted Hughes poem 'Full Moon and Little Frieda' came to mind: 'The moon has stepped back like an artist gazing amazed at a work that points at him amazed.'

Back with my neighbour on the pavement, I couldn't think of anything to say so I reverted to male stereotype: football. He supports Chelsea, so I managed to mouth some platitudes about how important the following weekend's games were for both of us.

But it was the sight of his baby that lingered in my mind. A gorgeous lump of loved flesh and spirit. That night in bed as I lay next to my partner, our bodies entwined, I mused. I pressed her hand and she pressed mine. There was no need for words. I am blessed to be with this amazing woman.

Is this the start of the healing?

Richard

I AM GODFATHER to our niece, who has recently given birth to her first child. We are now in touch with three small children and hear news of others in the extended family. So, we share in the joys and pain of the children, but always at a slight distance. I can listen to the conversations about child-rearing but never join in. When I'm with Laura's family I have a sense of not being fully adult. None of this is caused by anything said or done ... The sense of loss never completely goes away, though I can't say that this is a strong conscious and constant feeling; it's more one that comes and goes.

Aaron

AS THE YEARS have gone by, things have become easier and we now enjoy lots of time with our nieces, nephews and friends' children without it being an issue. We now find ourselves in a position of having lots of spare time and more available money to go and do fancy things which most of our friends do not. We have changed our social circle to those couples who do not have children or have children who are grown-up. I do miss some people that we spent a lot of time with, but a phrase we have in our house is that people come into your life for a reason, a season or a lifetime; and that seems about right. I now often find fathers envious of the life I have, which is ironic. I genuinely enjoy my life and now sometimes wonder if not having children has actually been a blessing. We are so lucky to be able to help our nieces and nephews, our parents and friends, and to be able to do so without having to consider other responsibilities first. Also being part of a male-only fertility support group has been great in that I have been able to provide that voice that life is OK if your fertility journey ends without children. It's not easy or nice at all, but there is a life to be had afterwards. I rather enjoy my life without children now; both for selfish reasons but also because we are now in a position to spontaneously help others out if they need it.

Shipwrecks and Sandcastles

NOTHING PREPARES YOU for Rhossili on the Gower penin-sula. A narrow, nondescript road winds between high hedges and scruffy trees bent double by centuries of gales. The eastern slope of the down is unremarkable and the pebble-dash houses that dribble along the outskirts of the village do nothing to hold the eye. Only as you round the corner by the tiny church, next to a field of untidy cabbages, does the full sweep of the bay come into view. Its impact is all the greater for having had no introductory fanfare. In 1957, when we first came here on holiday, I had seen nothing like it. I still know of few places to equal it. In this early autumn visit I needed to feel the deep joy of gazing on its three-mile-long beach, its clifftops, its hills and Worms Head. Even after a lifetime of travelling, it remains my favourite spot in the whole world. And maybe the fact that my ancestors on my mother's side were Welsh adds some piquancy.

It was here on a holiday when I was six that my soul woke up to nature. When I threw off the Home Counties mantle and discov-ered that the natural world could also be untamed and raw. Now I make the trip every two years or so. That time had come again.

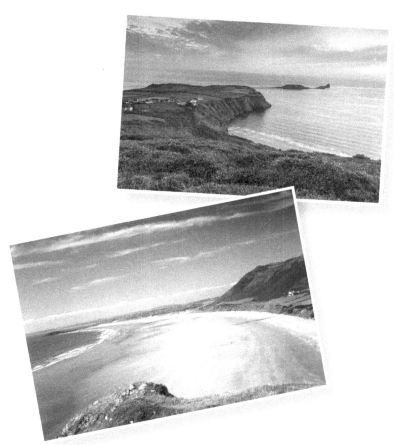

I don't know what it is about the view of the bay. Perhaps it's that you're several hundred feet above it at one end, while the outcrop of Burry Holms acts as a full stop to its arching sweep at the other. A geometrician might tell you that its curve is a perfect parabola. It may even be that the down and the haunted parsonage in the fields above the beach are in symbiotic union. All I know is that here I began to grow up.

I walked down the path to Rhossili beach and stopped at the wreck of the *Helvetia*, whose pock-marked timbers have been thrusting their gnarled shapes through the sand since 1887. It was here that the impoverished folk of Gower used to lure sailors ashore at night with lanterns, then attack them and steal their cargo. Much later, on this same swathe of sand, I used to play cricket with my father – our only boundaries the rim of the sea, the towering cliffs and the fading light.

These days, children with buckets and spades make sandcastles, and bronzed surfers use their boards to draw wiggly shapes in the sand on the long walk out to the waves. At the dunes, I turned inland towards the caravans at Llangennith. The floors of the shops here are covered in sand, thanks to the children who run in for flimsy fishing nets or colourful beach-balls.

Wind chimes tinkled on the breeze as I walked on and up the steep path of Rhossili Down, where heather and gorse blaze and the concrete foundations of Second World War gun turrets are still visible. At the top, hand gliders were floating like silent gulls and thin veils of cloud were sweeping in. The Pembrokeshire coast twinkled away to the west and, beyond the Loughor Estuary, the factories of Llanelli stood sullen and drab.

Back in Rhossili village, at the Worms Head Hotel where we used to stay, I picked out the window where I had hung up seaweed to predict the weather. 'Yes,' the receptionist said, 'Bill's still alive.' Bill had been the waiter. He used to hold the silver jug over your cup and then raise it two feet, pouring all the time to froth up the coffee. For years afterwards when we made coffee like that, we called it 'doing a Bill'.

In the gift shop there were no Toby jugs anymore. In the 1950s, I remember my sister and I had counted six different ways of spelling Rhossili on the base of those jugs. Now there was just one way.

The time had come to walk over to Worms Head. The tide was rolling back to reveal the magnificent sweep of the bay and a girl was driving cattle away from the cliff edge. The waters of the causeway over the Worms Head part like a Welsh Red Sea two hours before low tide. Apparently, the shape of its far-flung tip reminded the Vikings of the carved head of the dragon (or *wurm*) on the prow of their ships. The rocks soon emerge once the tide starts to recede. Over on the headland, I saw seals circling in the sea, two campers rolling a joint, and an Alsatian which came over and barked and snapped at my heels. As I always did, I looked for the blowhole in the rock, but once again I couldn't find it. I clambered onto the top of Worms Head, right at the end, where Dylan Thomas fell asleep in 1933 and had to wait overnight for the next low tide to get back.

Big grey clouds were rolling in from the west and the wind was getting up – it was bound to rain later. Oddly, I never remember it raining at Rhossili in the old days, but I'm sure it did. I remember the sunsets being golden, red, green and mauve, and how forked lightning lit up the down at night. Sure enough, all those years later, as I walked back over what seemed the bounciest grass in the world, the first drops of rain settled on my face.

This had been a happy journey back to the days of my childhood. Now, when I raised my head, I wasn't frowning. I was still childless but I didn't feel helpless and alone. Something must have breached my soul's defences.

Mike S

I BELIEVE I have accepted my childless state. Life is full of things I didn't expect, and in being childless I am not alone. I just get on with the life I do have and try to make the best of it. I think that can sometimes make me a little selfish but then I am missing so much that the majority enjoy, so I figure I'm going to do what I want to do. Sometimes it can almost make me feel privileged but in others I can feel cheated and envious. But, at the ripe old age of 64, I have much to be thankful for.

Jan

I HAVE ACCEPTED that I will never have children. It doesn't necessarily make things easier, though. Some days it still feels like an unbearable loss, a gaping hole in my life. Something I still mourn. I think I'm becoming more at peace with it, though. I have accepted it and it's part of me but it doesn't define me. I am also very aware that it allows me to live a life with enormous freedom, something I really appreciate. I recently met my niece and new-born nephew for the first time, while travelling overseas. I was quite nervous how it would make me feel but it was ok. Tough but ok. I was able to be happy on behalf of my sister and happy 'just' to be uncle. Part of my road to acceptance, perhaps?

So, What Now?

THERE YOU HAVE it: the pain and the anger, the hot hurt pouring from a cauldron of failed dreams. In that fire flicker the flames of all I hoped for as a fulfilled man, a grown-up citizen, a father. Those red and yellow shapes dance and mock me in my childlessness.

But that searing heat burns for everyone, whether man or woman, for failings of whatever kind. Failings that will never go away, failings that lie for ever at the centre of all that we are.

Then there are the wisps of disappointment drifting on the wind, the trailing remnants of youthful optimism.

Like all fires do, it subsides into a warm glow, giving us the chance to rake through the embers, to ruminate, to wonder why, to reflect and to analyse. The blaze dies down, but breezes fan those ashes back to life and the pain comes roaring back. Change is the one constant.

So, what now?

Is it all too late? Suddenly, as if in answer, the motley figures of some high-profile male celebrities who have fathered children late in life appear. They stand mischievously on my shoulder, smirking role models, and they set off in me a distinctly dubious train of thought.

I know, and I quake from feminists' wrath as I write this, that I could catch a plane to the Philippines tomorrow, meet a poor girl looking for a 'rich' Western man, get married within the month and maybe become a father within 12 months. Problem solved. A friend of mine did just that and the last I heard he was a happily married father of three, one of that large cohort of men, largely from the English-speaking world, who have taken this route. Some critics would say that this is an exotic form of exploitation. Earlier in this book I record an episode in which I, too, went to that same country to meet a girl, having spoken to her online, but the enterprise ended in failure. Perhaps I'd be luckier the next time.

Men do not have the menopause and can father children until their dying day, right? Hold on! It's not quite as simple as that, and here's why.

Firstly, contrary to popular belief, there is a male biological clock. A study by the Centre for Reproductive and Genetic Health found that the probability of a live birth drops by a third if the father is over 50. Stories of celebrity men fathering children in their sixties give a hugely skewed view.

Secondly, men produce sperm their whole life but the quality of that sperm, and therefore the chance of the woman conceiving, starts to go down from their twenties. And testosterone reduces from the age of 30, so in reality men become less fertile as they age. What's more, defective sperm increases the chance a child will be born with a disability.

When a couple is having difficulty conceiving, the medical profession invokes 'the rule of three' to try to find out the reason: the cause of the infertility is one third down to men, one third down to women and one third is unknown. So, the responsibility is more or less equally divided between the sexes, but the focus and the testing invariably fall on women.

Women wanting to increase their chances of having a baby readily make lifestyle changes such as giving up smoking, reducing their drinking and losing weight, but men usually do nothing. They think that because they ejaculate, they are producing healthy sperm but this is far from being the case. Besides, what they see is semen, not sperm; the latter being the all-important chemical ingredient.

So, I repeat: what now?

Sharing the unwanted grief of being childless with others in the same position and offering communal support is one way forward. The friendships that I have struck up with other men and women in the last few years have been so helpful in coming to terms with the issue. One group, The Childless Men's Community, has been particularly beneficial. And I hope I have been able to reciprocate on occasions. It is these men who have been the main contributors to the testimonies in this book. The way some of them have turned their fortunes round by reconfiguring their lives is inspirational. Such intelligent alleviation really does work.

The whole arena of childlessness is opening up for discussion, albeit by women for the most part. Jennifer Aniston's bold admission about trying for years to conceive with the help of IVF is just one example. Not least her acknowledgement that it was now too late, by saying that 'the ship has sailed'. In the men's arena, figures such as comedians Rod Silvers and Rhod Gilbert have added their thoughts to the debate.

But alleviation of the hurt doesn't really solve the problem. I need more than that. For weeks I couldn't think of a way to proceed. I couldn't write anything. This section of the narrative remained untouched as, again and again, I confronted the question I had posed for myself: what now? It was a case of 21st century writer's block. I had no answer to pronatalism's dominance. I wasn't part of it, so it had defeated me.

It will require courage to fill this space. I'm thrashing around not knowing which way to turn. A part of me wants to end here and leave everyone to their own devices, myself included. After all, I never set out to write a self-help book. As I wrote earlier, I am not a moral crusader, nor a therapist who believes that I can turn round people's lives.

So, that's it then.

But something still drives me on to forge a fragile permanence out of these smouldering, shifting remains. 'These fragments I have shored against my ruins', as TS Eliot has it in The Waste Land. I must barricade myself against despair and nihilism.

Perhaps all that's left is the quest for meaning, albeit a meaning that is ultimately unattainable. Don't be greedy, laddie. Don't ask for more: there isn't any. Just enjoy the search. Revel, if revel you will, in the dubious thrill of untangling the reasons why, when one wanted it so much, parenthood has evaded you. Season with contradiction and garnish with ambiguity and just eat the portion you've been given.

Be content with what you have. After all, you've got it pretty cushy: a white, middle-class male, living in the developed world, born in the second half of the 20th century. That's a privilege.

Then came other realisations. Not being a father has allowed me to do all sorts of things that I couldn't have done as a parent. I've travelled the world and been paid for glibly chatting about it on paper. Not bad. I've worked with clever people and with caring people. And I have had relationships with some amazing women, both beautiful and inspiring. What do I have to complain about? OMG I'm sounding disgustingly smug.

It was time to look longer and harder. This triggered a searing, honest assessment of myself. My amateur self-analysis underlined the bald, irrefutable fact that I do not have children, nor ever will. And that I have never married. Why had this eureka moment taken so long to hit me? These are facts. They can be accepted. They have to be accepted.

And, again, perhaps it is not just chance that has brought about this state of affairs. Perhaps there was, and is, something inescapable in my make-up that has created this. That, even given a different set of circumstances, it was always destined to end like this. Best to manufacture a peaceful accord with this failure. A kind of gentle, profound and sad Buddhist acceptance of the status quo. No need to set in motion a programme of deliberate transformation.

Another Buddhist trope is that we are forever changing, whether we like it or not. It is out of our control. So, to talk of the status quo is in fact misleading. This acceptance need not be static; it can be dynamic.

This is all freshly mined thought. I have no idea where it will lead. But I hear myself saying: do not turn away from the hurt but savour it. Ponder the creative potentialities of failure. Rake over the embers and new flames may leap from the ashes. By embracing the pain who knows what newness may creep into view?

Suddenly, there is great energy in this, an ecstasy of possibility even. It's quite feasible, then, to redefine oneself, to take a different path, to walk in the opposite direction. But those tired ideas that no longer serve a purpose need to be thrown away. A vibrant, youthful vision awaits – even as old age beckons.

I'm looking into the fire. Waiting.

Graham

IT IS DEFINITELY an acceptance now. I feel that I have processed grief and this has mainly been with the support of The Childless Men's Community'. The power that comes from being listened to by a group of non-judgemental, supportive and understanding men has been a great comfort. I've also shared openly my feelings with my wife's family and friends. I cannot really imagine myself with children now. I have a freedom that many would envy. I am living a great life and I'm healthy and happy. Just sometimes, there is something missing, but hey we can't have it all, can we?

Richard

THERE ARE ALSO benefits to being childless. I've been able to pursue my own interests. We don't have financial pressures and we can spend time together without the stresses and anxieties of being parents. Is this selfish? I don't think it's any more so than were our motives for wanting children. Of course, we don't have the joys and pleasures of children either, but in the end, though I do have regrets, I can't truly say that my life has been irredeemably damaged by being a childless man.

Childless Men's Testimonies

Can you describe the circumstances that led to you not being a dad?

Robin: I have four sisters so I couldn't do the objectifying/possession thing that I think other lads did. I was interested in girls as people and I don't think that attitude was seen as great back then. I got married and started trying for a baby but my wife, who was five years younger, started a new job with a younger crowd and decided she didn't need to become a mother yet. She was having too much fun. In my late twenties, we divorced. I bought out her half of the house, which was a big mistake because the housing market crashed. I couldn't sell and the mortgage payments were horrendous: I had only just enough money to meet the bills and eat. Then I got together with a younger woman, and we got on great. One day she said: 'I want to have your babies.' However, we split up soon afterwards. Then in my late thirties I met my wife who is a few years older than me. Although she had wanted to be a mum, now – because of the risks – she didn't want to go down that route. We discussed my wanting to be a dad and I had to make a choice. I chose love.

Mike S: My circumstances of not being a father follow a trag- ically failed surrogacy programme. My partner at the time was born with a rare condition where the womb does not develop, so conception is impossible. The only way to have a biological child of our own was host surrogacy. A suitable surrogate mother was identified and, following IVF treatment, she was pregnant with our child. Four months into the pregnancy she miscarried. It was the worst day of my life. UK law at the time insisted that parents of a surrogate child had to be married, so by then we were. My wife was so distraught I couldn't scrape her off the floor. Eventually we parted (completely without acrimony) and remain very close friends, meeting regularly still today. We did look at adoption but the experiences we had endured negated that option.

Do you ever feel lonely or depressed about not being a father?

John: Yes, absolutely. All of my friends have gone on to be fathers so I am definitely alone. I'm sad, too. Lots of the time.

Richard: I married my first wife, my girlfriend from school, when we were both 21. We were keen to travel and work overseas, and, when we had both qualified as teachers, we were about to leave for Africa when she became pregnant. She arranged an abortion (only recently legalised in the UK) then told me she'd done so, had the procedure at a down-at-heel south London clinic and we then flew out to Africa, all within about a 10-day period. Our marriage was already rocky and didn't ever recover, though we remained married (sometimes together, often apart) for another 10 years.

I met Laura when I returned to London after nearly a decade away. We were both on the rebound from relationships, supposedly a recipe for further failure, but we've been very happily married for 40 years. Having met in our early thirties though, the opportunity to have children was limited. Nevertheless, after four or so years together we tried for a child and she quickly became pregnant. She was almost at full-term when the baby died. Now it would be called a stillbirth, but then it was still a 'miscarriage'.

The medical staff had a brisk view – these things happen and you should just try again, as a GP friend of mine said. Looking back, I realise how traumatised we were, but we didn't seek help, nor was any offered. We didn't try again.

Though neither my brother or sister, both now dead, had children, Laura's brother and sister-in-law have a growing number of grandchildren and Laura's extended family is relatively large. In fact, I think that I miss my younger brother more, and the way we could have shorthand conversations, such as those around our shared passion for our local football club. He died of cancer in his early forties.

Andy: I am not alone as a childless man or as part of a childless couple – but it feels as if you are the only one due to the pronatal discourse that pervades our society. From sex education at school, getting a girl pregnant sounded as easy as looking at her – there were no words about the difficulties involved, the agony of miscarriages, the bizarreness of entering a room with a plastic pot – not being able to have children wasn't a reality shared. I had childless 'aunts' and 'uncles', friends of my parents, as invisible as I felt daily during our trying for children and on many occasions since. Yet I am not alone.

It is easy to become bitter, to create binaries of us and them – dominant privileged discourses invite this – but it doesn't help anyone, not us who suffer, nor parents. Pronatalism places expectations and pressures on us all to perform to norms we are never asked to question. Authenticity is lost all around. So, I place my energy elsewhere in co-creating community for childless men and people, in tackling discrimination. In essence, offering my desire to nurture, to nourish fellow childless people. For we are not alone, to borrow a phrase from a fellow childless man.

Mike S: I have never really grieved about being childless. I have never suffered depression or felt lonely either. I love people and make friends easily.

Mike C: Life without children at times feels like a process of having to justify one's existence. And I understand that. It makes complete sense that as a species here primarily to perpetuate ourselves, we would have in place codes and mores that would stigmatise childless-ness (surely the genesis – pun intended – of religious discrimination against same-sex relationships?).

Is it hard for you to be around families or men who are fathers?

Ken: There's been many times. Last year my wife's son and daughter came over. Her daughter with her boyfriend (her husband had passed away) came to celebrate my birthday. Shortly after they arrived, the conversation went to each of their kids. My wife has two, her son has two, her daughter has two, and of course her boyfriend has two. I sat there for a few minutes listening. Of course, I didn't have anything to add. I felt like a fool. I got so upset I had to leave the room. I felt like a nothing, a nobody, why was I here on earth? Why was I born?

Jason: One of the hardest things not to do is compare how you would do things differently, especially when I see dads who seem-ingly don't care about their kids. What I find helps is trying to take a step back, think about each person at more than just face value. They have something I would like, but just like me they may have multiple insecurities, regrets and things that 'would be so much better if only …'. I try to take stock of what I do have and the lives that I can have an impact on. No, I may not have children with whom I can have a lasting impact, but that does not stop me trying to benefit other people's lives.

Aaron: Not anymore. The only way in which I struggle still is that my brother does have children and therefore gets pretty much all the focus of my parents. They help out a lot and, when I do get to see them, they will then always talk about the grandchildren. Now I love my nieces very much, but I guess I feel that I have lost something with my parents as I didn't have children. I also wonder that, as my parents get older, I'll be the one to do all the caring and supporting them despite not getting the majority of their time over the last few years; we'll be seen as the ones with nothing to do.

Robin: Not so much now. They have their path and I have mine. I am jealous sometimes and tired of it at others. I am aware of how parents crowbar in that they are parents at every opportunity. I was at a psychology conference and the presenter described some behaviour and used pictures of his baby doing the task. There was an audible and felt 'coo' that made me narky. I thought: 'A room full of psychologists and they can't see that they are being played.' I was also jealous of the attention he received from the mainly female audience.

Do you find it difficult to talk about the feelings you have around not being a father?

John: I have difficulties talking to my wife about it. I think we are in different places in the process of grieving and accepting our loss and situation.

Has anyone said to you: 'You can always adopt, you know?'

Robin: I've always felt defensive about this question because, although I think I would have been a good dad – at least better than my dad – I'm not sure about being a good dad to an adopted child. We looked into it briefly but decided that our ages were against us and that my wife knew from her professional life that it is not easy and not a quick fix.

Sikhumbuzo: This comment kills me big time. It makes me feel incapacitated.

Aaron: I have lost count of the times we received advice about adopting. Quite frankly, it more often than not made me angry that people would try to brush over such an emotive subject with such a glib answer. I usually bit my tongue as the comments often came from people that did care about us but just didn't know what to say. I think this is probably one of the most hurtful times actually. When you feel that you are trying everything you can to have children and rather than being asked: 'How are you?', you're immediately given some kind of solution. All I needed was a beer and a chat.

John: I've been told I can adopt so many bloody times! Mostly it made me want to punch them in the nose! Like we hadn't thought of it! And like it's just something you do, easy peasy! Ugh, the ignorance.

Does being childless affect your social life and relationships?

Jan: Being in your mid-forties and without kids you are pretty much socially alienated. Moving to a new country made us realise how hard it is to find people to socialise with when you are childless. And we still deal with the grief, loss, sadness and gaping hole in our lives. We deal with it differently and it is still a source of conflict. People generally have absolutely no idea how incredibly tough and heart-breaking being childless is. I have received many hurtful comments over the years and I guess they mostly come out of simply not knowing or understanding. It has also negatively affected our relationships with our families.

Robin: My family are always posting about their children and grandchildren on social media. I noticed in my thirties how peers with kids would not include people without kids. That even happens on the street where we live. The kids connect the parents but the parents disconnect us. Yet quite often the kids are unsupervised and there seems to be an unspoken agreement that we all look after the kids but there is no quid pro quo for the childless.

Jason: Grieving for a life that hasn't been born is exactly how I would describe the feeling. Instead of grieving for a life lost, thinking about the moments enjoyed together, it's grieving moments that could have been.

After tests and an operation it was found out that I do not produce a particular hormone that creates sperm, so cannot have children of my own. My wife and I then spent another couple of years trying other methods, including IUI and adoption, without any luck. My wife found this period very difficult and feels like it's 'not meant to be', which I partially agree with but find it very difficult to accept. We are now trying our best to move on and live life to the fullest with the cards that have been dealt, using our circumstances to take risks that we couldn't have done if we had kids which I feel is very good for us both.

We tried to adopt. This was by far the most stressful time of our lives. The way we were treated was appalling and it all seemed to fall down because the person we dealt with didn't like my wife, Alicia. We were first told to cancel our request because we wouldn't be accepted because we supposedly did not earn enough money. As we run our own business, on paper it can be confusing for a typical nine-to-five council member to understand what we have coming in, but we certainly had more than enough income to support a family and we proved this. Through this process of poor communication Alicia was constantly having to chase them for any kind of feedback and support, even though it was promised that they were 'only a phone call or email away'. They then wanted to meet with us to 'tell us off' for picking them up on the faults they had made in the paperwork.

Basically, it was the first step in our realisation that all the adoption team wanted was yes-men who fitted neatly into their unrealistic box. We then moved on to the next stage, where after having a two-hour chat with us about our upbringing in which we detailed our lives up to the age of about 16, with no follow-up to discuss the rest of our lives and further adoption journey, we were again told to take ourselves out of consideration because 'you wouldn't be approved'. This was all because Alicia had some tough times as an early teenager and got a little upset when talking about them. No follow-up, no discussion about how that has developed her as a person and her outlook or how she would look toward her own children, just taking someone getting a little upset while talking about a traumatic experience way out of proportion and leading to the conclusion: 'you will not make good parents'. This is a very tough subject for us both but it was the main driver for us to try and take control back in our lives rather than have ill-informed people do it for us.

Aaron: We have changed our social circle due to not having children. We have had friends who tried to include us in their social lives but it was too tough. I didn't want to go to children's parties or even go out with friends who had children as they would constantly talk about them.

Mike S: Being childless has not adversely affected my social life to any great degree but I do occasionally struggle when with others who are parents. All they seem to want is to talk about what their children are up to and how they are progressing. I do have friends who are childless, either by design or otherwise, and I seem to relate to them much more easily and they appear to be more interested in me and what I'm doing. Subsequent relationships have been OK and I have now remarried and have a mature stepson. We get on very well but he has his own father and I will never be that person to him.

Do you feel that leaving a legacy is important?

Alastair: If I could continue the family name, that would be nice. But leaving a legacy is far more important. That's all about having an impact on the next generation, even if I don't know about it. We decided to sponsor a child to help them get a better chance in life.

If you were to become a father in the future, how would that make you feel?

Alastair: It would be fantastic. I remember walking with my wife through Florence saying that if we had a child, I wouldn't care what they wanted to do as long as they were happy. They could study art history in Europe, and we would fly over from Australia to see them whenever we could. As long as they were doing what made them happy.

Have you accepted the fact that you will never become a father? If so, how does that feel?

Aaron: I probably do have one or two occasions a year when the sense of 'missing out' hits me and can make me feel quite sad, but these are often short-lived feelings, and recently it's been tragedies that have given rise to this sadness. An example was last year with the passing of our 28-year-old nephew; a terribly sad event that raised emotions in me about not being a father and therefore never experiencing a parent's grief. I wonder if there are 'extra' highs and lows attached to emotions when you are parents and as childless men our emotional range is somewhat less? I'm not sure, but that's where my mind took me as I considered my sadness.

Jason: No, I haven't accepted being childless, but I don't think I ever will. I'm trying to look constantly at the positives like the children's lives I can have an impact on while also living a life with my wife that we wouldn't be able to live if we had kids and the responsibilities that come with that.

Russ: It is realisation and acceptance that the requirement to be a father was never about what I needed but what social norms have decided I must be. A quote I love to use is 'You don't choose a life, dad. You live one.' from the film *The Way*, spoken by Daniel (Emilio Estevez).

Graham: I think without realising and maybe subconsciously I have accepted my/our childless state. Acceptance of the above looks like contentment and a loss of the yearning that once was part of me. I met my soulmate and life partner who is childless at a point that my yearning had reduced significantly. For her, she had given up on the thought of a family before we met. We enjoy a 'freedom' not afforded to many friends with children and are able to make lifestyle and financial decisions more easily as we do not have the expense of raising children. We can and are spontaneous, taking holidays outside of school holidays. We are currently sorting out our wills. With this will come some sadness that our 'estate' will not be passed on to immediate family, however again secure in the knowledge that we can, if necessary, use equity release with little conscience. Underneath, there is sadness that we in effect met 'too late' and Mum does not have grandchildren. But maybe in these times of world uncertainty and climate crisis we should be applauded for not having children. Overall, I am content and in a happy place – childless.

The Facts

MEN AGEING WITHOUT a family are a large group within society but, despite this, very little research has been conducted up to now. Part of the reason is that the statistics, apart from in some Nordic countries, predominantly relate to women. However, research into male childlessness is finally taking place and is growing rapidly.

The academic researcher Dr Robin A Hadley has collected some interesting statistics relating to male childlessness in the UK. These include:

- 25 per cent of men over 42 are childless – this is approximately five per cent more than the figure for childless women within the same age group.
- 50 per cent of men who aren't fathers, but had wanted children, say that they have experienced isolation.
- 38 per cent of men who are childless not by choice have spoken of depression.
- 25 per cent of men who haven't had children but had wanted to say that they've felt anger.
- 56 per cent of men who had not had children but had wanted to state that they've been sad.

The reasons for childlessness amongst men

CHILDLESSNESS AFFECTS ONE in four men and one in five women over 45 in the Western world, according to the Organisation for Economic Co-operation and Development. And there is a similar level of yearning for parenthood amongst both childless men and women, which challenges the common idea that women are much more likely to want to have children than men.

There are many reasons why men might find themselves ending up childless. This could include life choices, class, child bereavement, economics, education level, gender, infertility, family break-up or relationship skills. The most significant issues that shape men's experience of unwanted childlessness include infertility and the timing of relationship formation and/or dissolution. In addition, there can be circumstantial reasons due to relationships – perhaps the man's partner didn't want children, changed her mind, was physically unable to have them, was postponing having them or experienced tokophobia (a fear of pregnancy and childbirth). Relationship breakdown is another common factor in male childlessness. The break-up of a long-term relationship in someone's mid-thirties has a greater negative impact on their chance of becoming a parent than if it happens to someone younger.

Infertility affects one in eight couples in the UK and around half of all infertility cases are due to the male partner. Men over the age of 35 typically experience a decrease in sperm health, which then goes on to affect pregnancy rates, time to conception, miscarriage risk, adverse pregnant outcomes and the health of offspring. It is a complex area and there is no definitive study on which all can agree. However, it is generally accepted that there is a decline in sperm quality of approximately 0.8 per cent from the age of 35, and then a further increase after the age of 45. The everyday environment (for example, men's lifestyle, heat, diet and stress) can all adversely affect sperm health. In particular, smoking is associated with a significantly reduced sperm count.

In contrast, some reasons can stem from childhood. For example, another factor that might be an indicator of childlessness later in life is an anxious childhood attachment. It has been found that people who are childless were significantly more likely to have developed an anxious attachment to their primary caregiver in childhood. If a child was unsure how their caregiver (usually their parent) was going to react, then this gets embedded in their expectations of relationships. The result is that that person may well be tentative in risking being rejected, mocked or embarrassed. Being shy is a good way of understanding how this phenomenon might play out in the reality of forming adult relationships.

There is a commonly accepted notion that men can become fathers at any age, but being an older dad is quite rare – fewer than two per cent of the men registered as fathers are aged 50 or over. For men who are not wealthy or famous, becoming an older dad is rarely an option. The stereotype of the older father denies reality and supports simple stereotypes that form traditional notions of men as invincible because they are always successfully virile.

The results of childlessness for men

THE MID-THIRTIES CAN be a time of particular frustration and anxiety for men who find themselves without children. Only when these men become fathers do they realise the source of their discomfort: it is then that they start to feel 'complete'. In contrast, men who remain childless may speak of a feeling of loss. These losses include the roles and social dividend associated with parenthood, family status and grandparenthood, and also a sense that there is something missing in their lives. In addition, while many childless men do not undergo medicalised fertility treatment to try to conceive a pregnancy with a partner, they report elements of complex bereavement and disenfranchised grief often associated with infertility and failed fertility treatment.

Childless people are often seen as 'available to care' and are 20 to 40 per cent more likely to provide support to their elderly parents than people with children.

Involuntarily childless people may be reminded of what they missed not just in mid-life, but also later in life. Older people are a hidden but significant population, with a current estimated population of one million aged 65 and over in the UK without an adult child to support them. The increase in men's life expectancies means that there will be more men without children who are living longer. It has been shown that relationships and social support are as important as physical health for well-being, and for preventing isolation and exclusion later in life. Older men are more likely to have very small networks, compared to women.

Older men are viewed, at best, ambivalently. In academic and professional discourse, older men are of little interest for three reasons. First, they are seen through the political-economic perspective and judged by being married, having a pension and being retired. Second, men tend to work, then die. Third, they are regarded as hard to reach and uncommunicative and therefore condemned by their non-participation. Grandparenthood is a social currency that non-grandparents cannot access.

Lone older childless men are often viewed as a threat and stereotyped as sexual predators. They are sometimes seen as 'dirty old men' and as 'sexually driven but also sexually inappropriate and/or sexually impotent', according to Dr Robin A Hadley in his book *How Is a Man Supposed to Be a Man?* An awareness of 'outsiderness' and a fear of being viewed as a paedophile are widely reported by men in this group.

The older childless also tend to have smaller social networks than the equivalent aged parents. They therefore find it difficult to access informal care. A report by the Institute for Public Policy Research predicted that by 2030 there will be over two million childless people aged 65 and over without an adult child to support them. Some 20 per cent of these people will need 20 hours' care a week from someone who is not a relative. The consequences for government health and social care provision are huge. Men who reach old age as a single, childless adult therefore invariably worry about how they will finance good quality health and social care services in the absence of family members who may have otherwise been able to care for them. Social care policy does not appear to take the needs of childless older people into account at present. In terms of recognition, childlessness and grandchildlessness may deny older individuals a crucial buffer to the prejudice and discrimination associated with older age.

My thanks to one person in particular who has contributed the overwhelming part of the information – Dr Robin A Hadley, the leading academic writing on male childlessness.

Resources and Support

THERE ARE A large number of resources for childless women but very few specifically for childless men. I have endeavoured to list as many of these as possible. Some organisations' material will be equally relevant to both men and women. (These listings are correct at the time of publication.)

Organisations/Online Support

The Childless Men's Community: a closed Facebook men-only group giving support to childless-not-by-choice males. *facebook. com/groups/childlessmenscommunity*

The Full Stop Community CIC: an online support and network hub with a monthly podcast and online, diverse community open to all who identify as childless not by choice. *thefullstoppod.com*

Ageing Without Children: a campaigning group that provides information and support. *awwoc.org*

Gateway Women: a support and advocacy network, with a section devoted to childless men. *gateway-women.com/resources/resources-for-men*

World Childless Week: an annual event that offers support for childless-not-by-choice men and women. *worldchildlessweek.net*

Childless Not by Choice: a Facebook group offering support to the childless. *facebook.com/groups/591443651208173/members*

Married and Childless: a blog by a married Australian couple offering support. *marriedandchildless.com* and *www.thefullstoppod.com*

Walk in Our Shoes: men's and women's experiences of living the childless-not-by-choice life. *walkinourshoes.net*

Dr Robin A Hadley: a website with helpful resources from the world's leading academic on male childlessness. *robinhadley.co.uk/childlessness*

James D'Souza: a counselling website to help men dealing with infertility and childlessness. *jamesdsouza.com*

The Dovecote Community: a closed Facebook men-only group offering support to the childless. *facebook.com/groups/thedovecotecommunity4men*

Mensfe: men's fertility forum providing information and support. *mensfe.net*

Men's Fertility Support Group: a closed Facebook men-only support group for infertile men. *facebook.com/groups/mensfertilitysupport*

Fertility Network: support for those living without children due to infertility. *fertilitynetworkuk.org/life-without-children*

Happy and Childless App: an app offering friendship for the childless. *happyandchildless.co.uk/happy-and-childless-app*

Books

Dr Robin A Hadley (2021) *How Is a Man Supposed to Be a Man? Male Childlessness – a Life Course Disrupted*. Berghahn Books

Bruce Gillespie and Lynne Van Luven (editors) (2008) *Nobody's Father: Life Without Kids*. TouchWood Editions

Rob Hutchings (2021) *Downriver Nomad: A Triathlete's Adventures and Adversities into the Rapids*. Rob Hutchings

Mary-Claire Mason (1993) *Male Infertility – Men Talking*. Routledge

Lorna Gibb (2019) *Childless Voices: Stories of Longing, Loss, Resistance and Choice*. Granta Books

Steve Petrou (2018) *I Only Wanted to be a Dad: A Man's Journey on the Road to Fatherhood*. VASPX Publishing

Elliot Jager (2015) *The Pater, My Father, My Judaism, My Childlessness*. The Toby Press

Glenn Barden (2014) *My Little Soldiers*. Piranha Press

Articles

Sirin Kale. 'I'm scared I've left it too late to have kids: the men haunted by their biological clocks'. *theguardian.com/lifeandstyle/2021/oct/28/scared-late-kids-men-biological-clocks-ageing-procreation-anxieties*

Bibi Lynch. 'Male childlessness: 'You think, If I'm not reproducing – then what am I?' *theguardian.com/lifeandstyle/2018/nov/17/male-childlessness-not-reproducing-what-am-i*

Dr Robin A Hadley. 'I know all about broody men who long to be dads. I am one.' *telegraph.co.uk/men/relationships/fatherhood/9969542/Robin-Hadley-I-know-all-about-broody-men-who-long-to-be-dads.-I-am-one*

Dr Robin A Hadley. 'Male broodiness: Does the desire for fatherhood affect men?' *zenodo.org/record/4296637#.ZFjLrnbMK3A*

Media

My Name is Rod: a podcast featuring Rod Silvers talking about male infertility. *bbc.co.uk/sounds/play/m00066zc*

Rhod Gilbert: Stand Up to Infertility: a TV programme in which the comedian Rhod Gilbert brings awareness to male fertility issues. bbc.co.uk/programmes/p0957848

Childless Not By Choice: a US podcast containing episodes focusing on male childlessness. *childlessnotbychoice.net*

England Expects (2011): a short, humorous film about IVF set against the background of the World Cup. *youtube.com/watch?v=xMRTXi6uMAE*

Terry and Jude (2018): a play that raises issues around male childlessness. *acebook.com/GameOfTwoHalvesProductions*

The Easy Bit (2019): a full-length film in which six men talk honestly about their fertility treatment. *youtube.com/watch?v=__UDktJ_1c0*

Printed in the USA
CPSIA information can be obtained
at www.ICGtesting.com
LVHW062229150923
758322LV00015B/159